EBURY PRESS
TALKING TO THE BABY IN THE WOMB: GARBHA VIDYA

Dr S. Bhaskar and Dr S. Andal Bhaskar established Dr. Andal's Lakshmi Fertility Clinic in 1989 in Nellore, Andhra Pradesh, and the clinic is now a leading centre for first-class medical care in infertility, obstetrics and gynaecology. Till date, they have successfully treated thousands of patients with infertility and Dr Andal Bhaskar has helped more than 10,000 mothers deliver.

Over the years, Dr Andal Bhaskar has combined ancient Indian wisdom with her own experience to develop special techniques that a modern mother-to-be can use to not just have a normal delivery but create an emotional bond with the baby even before birth. The couple has been offering these techniques at their clinic in Nellore. Together, they have conducted patient education programmes in their clinic for the past thirty-six years and have also been educating the public through their YouTube channel—Andal Fertility Channel—which contains more than 1295 videos that have been well received by the public.

Dr Andal Bhaskar, an alumnus of Stanley Medical College, Chennai, and Kurnool Medical College, Andhra Pradesh, has several international papers and publications to her credit.

Apart from the English edition, this book is also available in Hindi, Telugu, Tamil and Kannada. Regional language books are available on amazon.in.

For long-distance patients, online consultations are available. For more details, contact +919908854316, +919440278177, 0861-2327018.

YouTube: https://www.youtube.com/c/andalfertilitychannel

PRAISE FOR THE BOOK

'It is indeed a proud privilege to have the opportunity to write about *Talking to the Baby in the Womb: Garbha Vidya*, so painstakingly written by Dr Andal Bhaskar of Nellore.

I got an opportunity to visit Nellore for a lecture. I went to the hospital run by Dr Andal and her husband Dr Bhaskar and listened to a school headmistress, who had come from Kuwait and had delivered at their hospital. It was her second delivery. During the interaction, she said, "I enjoyed my delivery." It was a big surprise for me to hear a patient talking about "enjoying" a delivery. This opened a new line of thought for me. With *Talking to the Baby in the Womb*, this "new" and "old" approach will reach many practitioners of modern medicine and thereby benefit numerous would-be mothers. I have used the words new and old approach because this is an age-old Indian tradition that has to be learnt afresh.

I strongly recommend *Talking to the Baby in the Womb* to each and every person connected with the welfare of women. With its focus on relationship and confidence-building, the book will help in bringing down the incidence of caesarean section, not only in India but all over the world. Combining modern medicine with love, care, affection and self-confidence is a step in the right direction. In fact, when I heard a woman say that she had enjoyed her delivery, I could not believe her. When I put the same question to many of my relatives, they confirmed that they, too, had enjoyed the experience of pregnancy and childbirth. For a practitioner of modern medicine, which mainly focuses on linear (reductionist) thinking, some of the parts will take time to be accepted. Those exposed to non-linear (holistic) thinking will accept and apply these principles much faster.

Talking to the Baby in the Womb is a step in the right direction. I do hope and trust that Dr Andal's well-wishers and admirers in India and abroad will wholeheartedly support her. The initiative of Happy Delivery (Anandi Balantapan) in Pune has its seeds in Nellore. I wish Dr Andal and Dr Bhaskar all the very best in their endeavour to make pregnancy and childbirth a humane experience to be cherished forever'—**Dr Shirish Patwardhan, MD, president, Pune Obstetric and Gynecological Society (2012–13); president, Association of Maharashtra Obstetric & Gynaecological Societies, 2010–12; senior vice president, Federation of Obstetric and Gynecological Societies of India (FOGSI), 2009; and chairperson, Safe Motherhood Committee, FOGSI, 2003–07**

'[In] *Talking to the Baby in the Womb: Garbha Vidya* [Dr Andal Bhaskar] has given practical advice coupled with wisdom to all pregnant women.

I hope that the perusal of this book will guide many a pregnant woman to enjoy their pregnancy and child rearing'—**Dr P. Balamba, PMD, DGO, consultant obstetrician and gynaecologist, Shalini Hospitals**

'When we read this book we are often reminded of the happenings in the lives of the famous epic persons like Abhimanyu and Prahalad, etc. We studied these things in our school days. We read that these epic people learnt several things while they were in their mother's womb and they acquired their great qualities of courage, confidence, decision-making and more. In this book, Dr Andal Bhaskar has proved scientifically that it is possible to develop the right psychology in babies while they are in the mother's womb. In this modern age, every family can follow and practise such techniques to deliver healthy, happy, intelligent and confident babies. She has given several examples from her experience in the medical profession.

In every family, if the parents can practise the "talking to the baby" methods suggested by Dr Andal, then their children will become intelligent, courageous, self-confident and acquire a good personality. Such children would be able to withstand all the troubles they face in the present society with confidence and will be successful. They would be able to solve any difficult problems by themselves without depending on others. Such children are an asset to the family, and they contribute to the peace and harmony of society and of the nation. Then our nation will prosper through their contributions. So, in every family, parents must read this book, and they must encourage others to read it. They have to practise the methods suggested in this book and achieve good results.

I congratulate Dr Andal Bhaskar for putting into practice her thoughts and ideas through her clinic and encouraging the parents to follow her methods and getting good results during the last three decades. I wish that Dr Andal brings many more such scientific writings and methods and contribute to the prosperity of our society and nation. I encourage all parents to read this book'—V. Veeraiah, PhD, former vice chancellor, **Vikrama Simapura University, Sri Potti Sriramulu, Andhra Pradesh**

'The work *Talking to the Baby in the Womb: Garbha Vidya: Ancient Wisdom for Modern Mothers* by Dr Andal Bhaskar is a groundbreaking point of departure with the common understanding of foetal science. The text draws attention to primarily three things: the first is the elaboration of ancient wisdom regarding Indian eugenics, the second is its close affinity with modern science, and the third is its perennial relevance in terms of applicability and association with *every* time and zone of the human world. The text has dared to endeavour the recesses of ancient modernity of Talking to the Baby in the Womb by unravelling the "mythos" part of Indian scriptural tradition, which seldom gets contextualized to the depth of common.

In addition, it also gives spatial ground to modern experiences (with careful liberty I would regard them as "experiments") of many public personalities in terms of the application of this ancient science. The significance of the father along with the mother in the shaping of one's unborn child and their role in the formation of her future is also presented with attentive care and verbal simplicity. Apart from that, how the simple mode of storytelling (which actualizes the Indian mode of transmitting knowledge) designs the early layers of consciousness. And how the internal dialogue of mother with her child in the womb affects the post-birth cycle of habit formation is also explicitly framed in a highly illustrative and subtle narrative. The connection among the chapters and simplicity of medium are also what make this book a must-read for all parents.

For long, my interest in the area of prenatal care and education has propelled me to inspire and remain in accordance with the scholars diligently working in this field and as a head of the only university across the world working in this area, I feel greatly rejuvenated and energized with the advent of this path-breaking text by Dr Andal Bhaskar. I extend my warm wishes to her for undertaking this scholarly expedition with missionary zeal and academic temerity and cannot resist myself to urge her to continue the chain with more studies following this trail'—**Prof. D.K.S. Likhiya, former vice chancellor, Children's University, Gandhi Nagar**

'This is a beautiful book. For the precious nine months that you carry your baby within you, both can experience an intimacy that will envelop you right through your lives as mother and child.

The book is based on Dr Andal's thirty-plus years of "hands-on" and "mind on" research with prospective mothers, during pregnancy and soon afterwards. While most mothers instinctively know that their babies feel their moods and feelings, many are not immediately confident of Talking to the Baby in the Womb.

Dr Andal has used a lovely fictional style to get her message across.

The synthesis of science, faith and spirituality is evident in this book. The role of the husband, family and even social interaction is explored. Music and its magical powers are called into play. You will enjoy the book and will be able to pass on this knowledge to your children in the years ahead. I wish you the joy of being a mother, which is the greatest experience given to humans'—**Dr Rekha Shetty, managing director, Mindspower, and author**

'In one line: Every family must own this book. This book has to be translated in all languages, for the benefit of the present and future generations.

I have been associated with Dr Andal and her team for the last ten years. This book is an answer to all the questions that are likely to arise in a prospective parent's mind. Dr Andal has addressed this issue of suffering and how we can overcome them through simple steps of mind- and body-related interventions.

Dr Andal has distilled her decades of experience in treating prospective parents and brought out her wisdom in this book. This book is in a narrative form, full of metaphors, analogies and examples, which any common man can easily decode the technical factors behind each of the issues handled. She has gone into the ancient times much before the modern medical world of chemicals came into origin, and dug out lessons of the impact of society, relations and a sense of security that those days offered to young couples and she linked it with the modern world of medicines and offered innovations to help these young couples who might be missing such a compassionate family togetherness.

This book also provides support to medicos engaged in the sphere of fertility, pregnancy, antenatal support, with lot of useful tips about coping behaviour of their patients.

Fortunate to have this book in my hand'— **R. Gopinath, CEO, Gopast Centre for Learning; managing director, Harmoney Wealth Advisory Services India; and former CEO and managing director, LIC Lanka**

TALKING TO THE BABY IN THE WOMB

GARBHA VIDYA

Ancient Wisdom for Modern Mothers

DR S. ANDAL BHASKAR
DR S. BHASKAR

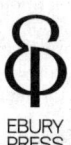

EBURY PRESS

An imprint of Penguin Random House

EBURY PRESS

Ebury Press is an imprint of the Penguin Random House group of companies whose addresses can be found at global.penguinrandomhouse.com

Published by Penguin Random House India Pvt. Ltd
4th Floor, Capital Tower 1, MG Road,
Gurugram 122 002, Haryana, India

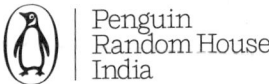

First published in Ebury Press by Penguin Random House India 2025

Copyright © Dr Andal Bhaskar and Dr S. Bhaskar 2025

Illustration copyright © Senthil Kumar

All rights reserved

10 9 8 7 6 5 4 3

The statements, opinions and strategies expressed in this book are based on the authors' own study and research and the publisher assumes no liability for the same. The publisher and the author provide no warranties of any kind with respect to this book's contents, any line of healthcare, treatment or diet. This book is for informational purposes only and is not intended to diagnose, treat, cure, or prevent any condition or disease. It is not intended as a substitute for professional medical advice, diagnosis, or treatment, which must be undertaken under the direction of a healthcare provider or physician. Neither the author nor the publisher shall be liable or responsible for any loss or adverse effects allegedly arising from any information or suggestion in this book. While every effort has been made to ensure the accuracy of the information presented, neither the authors nor the publisher assumes any responsibility for errors. References are provided for information purposes and do not constitute an endorsement of any sources, drugs or medicines.

Please note that no part of this book may be used or reproduced in any manner for the purpose of training artificial intelligence technologies or systems.

ISBN 9780143476924

Typeset in Sabon LT Std by Manipal Technologies Limited, Manipal
Printed at Thomson Press India Private Limited

This book is sold subject to the condition that it shall not, by way of trade or otherwise, be lent, resold, hired out or otherwise circulated without the publisher's prior consent in any form of binding or cover other than that in which it is published and without a similar condition including this condition being imposed on the subsequent purchaser.

www.penguin.co.in

This book is dedicated to our beloved parents and in-laws, who are blessing us from heaven and driving us forward in doing this special work.

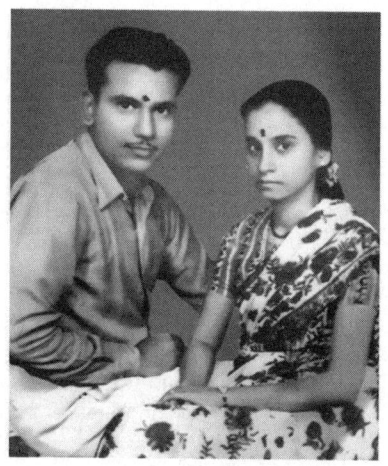

*Sri Chinni Krishnan and
Smt. Hemalatha*

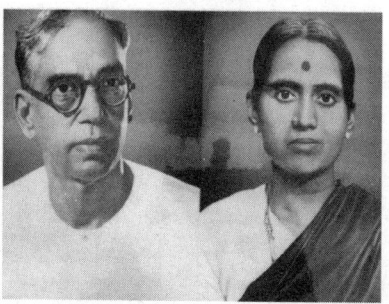

*Sri S. Balasundaram and
Smt. S. Lakshmi Bai*

Contents

Foreword — xv
Authors' Note — xvii
Introduction — xxi

1. The Technique and Concept of Talking to the Baby in the Womb — 1
2. Hope, Courage and Confidence — 33
3. The Significance of the Father's Role — 62
4. Intelligence — 84
5. Behaviour Modification — 109
6. The Tunes of Life — 131
7. Sports — 154
8. Happy Helpers in Reducing Nausea and Vomiting — 171
9. Meditation and Yoga — 187
10. Nutrition and Diet — 213

Acknowledgements — 245
Annexure and FAQs — 249
Testimonials — 263

Foreword

Dr. Kiran Bedi
Lieutenant Governor

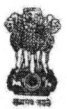

Raj Nivas
Puducherry 605 001
Phone : 0413 2334050
Fax : 0413 2334025
E-mail : lg.pon@nic.in

February 25, 2020

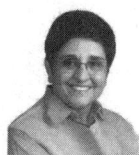

MESSAGE

I am extremely pleased to note that Dr. S. Andal Bhaskar, has authored the book entitled "TALKING TO THE BABY IN THE WOMB, that narrates in detail how to communicate with the baby in the womb.

Dr. S. Andal Bhaskar, practising Gynaecologist for more than 25 years and having done more than 10,000 deliveries has chronicled the knowledge and experience gained from her experience on how the right habits practised by mothers of reading scriptures, listening to music and helping themselves to be in a happy environment, produced good and intelligent children.

I am confident that this book will be a treasured and valuable document in the hands of 'mothers to be'. By practising what has been written in the book, the mothers can produce and nurture children who will be good human beings and contribute to the cause of nation building.

I convey my best wishes for the successful launch of the book.

(DR. KIRAN BEDI)

Authors' Note

The aim of this book is to allay the anxiety and fear of the pregnant mother and to aim at bringing a great personality on to this earth by virtue of her thoughts and talking to the baby in the womb.

The pregnant mother is the interface between the external world and baby. What mother eats nourishes the child; mother's oxygen is baby's oxygen; what mother thinks, each thought releases some chemicals that affect the mother, but as baby is connected to the mother through the umbilical cord, the blood with chemicals also reaches the foetus in utero and produces the same influence in the child. If the mother is happy, child will be happy.

Subconscious mind is highly developed in the child in the womb and continues to be predominant till the age of six. Ninety per cent of ours is subconscious and all activities in the body like regulation of heart and all other organs are managed by it. It is action-oriented and whatever is recorded is executed. So, the mother's thoughts during pregnancy play a major role in forming the subconscious mind of the foetus such that they are executed with precision later.

If the mother is stressed, or unhappy throughout pregnancy, stress hormones produced in the mother affect the child in the womb with adverse outcomes and disturbed behaviour of the child.

As a part of decreasing fear and anxiety during pregnancy and labour, we have initiated a technique of bonding with the baby in the womb. We ask our mothers to talk to the baby in the womb. Eventually, we have seen the mother becoming more confident, delivering without much complication in these cases. We also observed that the child has been responding to the mother as they have talked.

The whole process has been explained in the book. Feedback from the mothers about their experiences has been given in different chapters of the book.

Every mother irrespective of caste, colour, creed, religion, educated/ uneducated, rich/poor, with power/ without power has got the capacity to imagine and visualize the qualities of the child she is going to have. This is a power given by God/Nature to every woman to produce a child of the highest calibre, which she desires. Whole of the book explains of how to go about that.

Our dream is that if every woman/mother gets this information and knowledge that she is the creator of her own destiny, she will be able to give birth to the best quality human beings as no mother longs to have a bad person as her child. They should know for sure that they can have a hand in sketching the personality of the child, not just intelligence but also behaviour. It in turn, gives a good human being to society. Despite society playing different influences, the mother's effect is strongly imprinted in the subconscious mind of the child.

Let us try to bring in a society just by passing this information to every pregnant mother, such that in the time to come, we may have an evolved, and peaceful society. Most of the destruction in the world at present is due to distorted human behaviour where changes can't be brought by law and order.

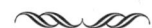

Introduction

Dear pregnant mother,

Hello! Welcome to the wonderful world of motherhood. Pregnancy is a blessing, and you are in for an amazing experience. With thirty-plus years of experience in gynaecology and obstetrics, and having delivered over 10,000 babies successfully, I want to take you through a special aspect of pregnancy and beyond.

You may be wondering, 'What is so special about the practice of an obstetrician? It's just the age-old mechanical job of delivering babies, except that the scene of action is hospital instead of home'. You are partly right; however, there is more to it than what meets the eye. Let me give you an analogy.

A jeweller looks at a gold bangle and values it only as gold. A person with an artistic bent of mind looks at it as 'a bangle with intrinsic design.' This analogy tells us that our perception of things makes the reality different.

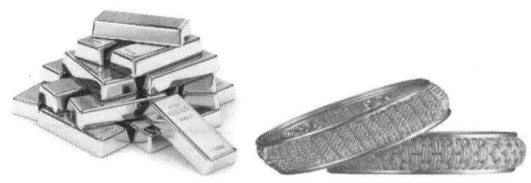

We see things not the way they are, but the way we perceive. Similarly, pregnancy is not just carrying and delivering babies; it is more than that. Let me narrate how my personal experiences and introspection changed my perception, from seeing just gold, to beautiful gold bangles. The mother's feelings influence the course and outcome of the pregnancy in both positive and negative ways. In my several years of practice, I found two situations intriguing.

- One, minor physical ailments, surprisingly, not responding well to medical treatment and keep recurring, such as recurrent UTI (urinary tract infection), tightness of abdomen, back pain, etc.
- Two, high-risk pregnancy with problems—contrary to expectation, in some cases, the course of pregnancy is smooth with successful outcome.

When I closely followed the details of such situations, I noticed the impact of mind over body. When the mental attitude was positive, medical treatment was effective. When there is even an iota of doubt or negative belief, state-of-the-art (high-tech) treatment proves ineffective. The reason: our emotions control hormones. Joy, happiness, feeling secure and positive beliefs trigger happy hormones like beta endorphin and serotonin. These hormones reinforce the body function, making the treatment more effective. Guilt, anxiety, doubt and negative beliefs trigger a stress hormone called cortisol. These hormones cause physical effects in the body such as increasing blood sugar, blood pressure, recurrent infections, etc.

Here, let me correlate the power of reassurance given by our ancestors to prevent anxiety and expect positive outcome by repeating proverbs such as 'The one who planted the seed, will surely water it'. Such positive attitude has acted as an effective medicine in the past and helped our great-grandmothers handle pregnancies easily.

Pregnancy has emotional, physical, mental and sensory aspects. A healthy coordination of all four is important to make it a pleasant experience. I can assure you that there is a simple way to get them right. The method evolved slowly through observation of expectant mothers, reading, analysis, discussion, applying and seeing the results.

How to Make Our Treatment Successful

These days people want to know the 'why' of the disease and strongly believe that medicine is a sure cure and want it only as a sugar-coated pill. I have understood the need to clear their doubts, instil confidence in a palatable way and give treatment. Let me explain the evolution of the method.

I observed two common concerns among expectant mothers:

1. Fear about delivery pain
2. Fear about baby's well-being.

I felt the need to empower the mother to overcome fear; this would help make the treatment effective. As I had been observing mothers during delivery, I could clearly see their anxiety, helplessness and insecure feeling during the course of labour. When they gave up and felt, 'I can't do it any more', labour used to come to a standstill, i.e. cervix, the mouth of the womb, stopped dilating further (cervical dystocia). On the contrary, when the delivering mother was relaxed and happy, it opened up easily.

Once during a delivery, when the cervix stopped dilating at 6 cm (full dilatation is 10 cm), I asked the woman if anything was bothering her. She replied she wanted her husband to be with her and he was on duty; I immediately spoke to him to get permission to be with her for a short while. When he came, we allowed him to be with her, ensuring privacy. After one hour, she was relaxed and smiling; to my surprise, the cervix had fully dilated and she delivered easily. This incident was an eye-opener that made me understand that if the pregnant mother is well prepared during pregnancy, she will definitely go through labour easily.

I started my initiative, approaching the husband and parents to extend moral support to the expecting mother. The family members didn't seem to understand the concept. They said, 'She is not tense or stressed. She is free and there is no pressure from us; we look after her very well.' When I asked them how they encourage her, they said, 'Yes, we keep telling her not to worry'. I told them, it's better to say, 'I'm with you. You will do well during delivery.' It was obvious that they were not used to uttering such encouraging words and were not willing to change their ways. I then felt that we, doctors and medical staff, need to be supportive. We planned to create a homely atmosphere in the hospital so that the expecting mother may feel relaxed. This was helpful to a certain extent.

Birth of Talking to the Baby in the Womb

In pursuit of an effective technique to make the expecting mother happy and confident, I discussed with other doctors and sociologists and read books. I stumbled upon this technique of Talking to the Baby in the Womb, while treating an expecting mother. She was originally from north India and didn't know the local language, Telugu; she used to come alone for check-up, as her husband was a busy executive. I was surprised to see her happy and relaxed without any complaints. On enquiry, I learnt she was talking to her baby in the womb and was enjoying the company! That was the secret of her confidence.

This was my eureka moment!

I had found the right technique of making expecting mother happy and confident. As I was sharing these observations with others, my brother insisted that I write a book on these experiences for the benefit of society. In the process of writing my experiences, I explored scientific studies to support my approach and I came across Dr Thomas R. Verney, Dr Chamberlain, Dr Bruce Lipton and Dr Deepak Chopra who have done pioneering work in the area of prenatal psychology.

Dr Thomas Verny was the first person to collect evidence worldwide of the effects of bonding of mother and baby during pregnancy and wrote *The Secret Life of the Unborn Child* with John Kelly. Later, with more evidence, he wrote *Pre-Parenting*. Dr Bruce Lipton wrote *The Biology of Belief* and Dr Chaberlain, *The Mind of Your Newborn Baby*. With the enormous experience in their path-breaking work, they all recommend conscious parenting as a harbinger of a peaceful and happy family and society.

I could see the wealth of information. These scientific studies are accessible to scientists, but the beneficiary is the lay public. How can they avail the information and translate it into action? I was thrilled as I was holding the key to the treasure trove. Yes! Talking to the Baby in the Womb is the key to conscious parenting; every conscious parent can use it to bond with her unborn baby and chart its path to sure health, happiness, intelligence and good qualities. Being an obstetrician, I have had first-hand experience of watching both the magic and tragic effects of the mother's mental state on the baby.

Let us briefly see what these pioneers have to say about research studies of bonding during pregnancy. Bruce Lipton says,

Your children's genes reflect only their potential, not their destiny. It is for you to provide the environment that allows them to develop the highest potential. Genes account for 49% of the factors that determine IQ and 51% of child's potential intelligence is controlled by environmental factors. Parents have a choice. They can fully reprogramme their limiting beliefs about life before they bring a child into their world. Research shows that if the mother is under stress, the baby's blood preferentially flows to arms and legs, causing babies to be born smaller and suppress forebrain function. Providing, nurturing pre and perinatal environment as well as good nutrition at crucial point in child's development results in blossoming of wonderful children. For human beings the most potent growth promoter is not the fanciest school, the biggest toy or the highest paying job. For human babies and adults, the best growth promoter is Love. How much better to become conscious parents and wonderful role models so that your children and their children will be conscious parents making for a happier and more peaceful planet.*

Let us see what Dr Thomas Verny says in *Secret Life of the Unborn Child*:

---

* Lipton, Bruce. *The Biology of Belief: Unleashing the Power of Consciousness, Matter and Miracles* (Penguin Random House India, 2016), pp. 144–51.

We now know that the unborn child is an aware, reacting human being, who from the sixth month on (and perhaps even earlier) leads an active emotional life. Along with this startling finding, we have made these discoveries:

- Most importantly, he can feel—not with an adult's sophistication, but feel nonetheless.
- Whether he ultimately sees himself and, hence, acts as a happy or sad, aggressive or meek, secure or anxiety—ridden person depends, in part, on the message he gets about himself in the womb.
- The chief source of those shaping messages is the child's mother. Chronic anxiety or a wrenching ambivalence about motherhood can leave a deep scar on an unborn child's personality.
- New research is also beginning to focus much more on the father's feelings. They show that how a man feels about his wife and unborn child is one of the single most important factors in determining the success of a pregnancy.

With this new knowledge at their disposal, mothers and fathers have an unparalleled opportunity to help shape the personality of their unborn child and contribute to his happiness and well-being, and not just in utero, nor in the years immediately following birth, but for the rest of his life.*

---

* Verny, Thomas with Kelly, John. *The Secret Life of the Unborn Child* (Dell, 1981).

Now we understand that baby's personality can be effectively shaped during pregnancy by the mother and father, and that Talking to the Baby in the Womb is an easy and sure way to achieve it. When we admire the efforts and knowledge of these western pioneers for enlightening the concept, we can't help but wonder at the amazing wisdom of our ancestors in observing and recording such facts about icons like Prahalada and Abhimanyu in our ancient Puranas. The possibility was observed in the past and proved in the present.

Personality, Prahalada

The story of Prahalada is a perfect example for understanding the making of a personality. Although Prahalada was the son of a Rakshasa (demon), who considered Lord Vishnu his archenemy, Prahalada came into the world as a staunch devotee of Lord Vishnu. By nature, Prahalada carried the genes of Rakshasa (hatred). The nurturing words of Sage Narada during pregnancy made him develop behaviour completely in contrast to his genetic makeup. He blossomed into a great devotee of Lord Vishnu. This was possible only because of Talking to the Baby in the Womb.

Knowledge and Skill

The case of Abhimanyu, the valorous son of Arjuna, is an ideal example. He listened to Arjuna's narration of the strategy to break into Chakravyuha (Padmavyuha) in the womb and retained the knowledge even as he grew up. He could remember the technique so well, even after so many years, he was able to break the Chakravyuha in Kurukshetra.

I was initially advising Talking to the Baby in the Womb technique to allay the anxiety of the expecting mother. When correctly followed, the bonding with the baby makes her happy; her anxiety and fear disappear, just like darkness vanishing in the presence of light.

The once drooping, anxiety-ridden face becomes bright with smiles. She is at ease and eagerly shares her experience of bonding with the baby; how confidently and easily she is able to carry on her work and able to brush aside horror stories told by others. This magic has to be seen to be believed. This gives our whole team immense happiness and energy boost to work more.

As I started promoting Talking to the Baby in the Womb to mothers, I observed mothers becoming positive and got feedback on the effect it has on the baby after birth. Mothers with strong intentions, found their children having the very qualities they desired during pregnancy. Similarly, anxious mothers' babies were jittery and restless, reflecting their womb environment. The dual benefits of Talking to the Baby in the Womb are happy, confident mother and well-groomed baby. It's like sowing good-quality seed (during pregnancy) in fertile soil (womb) and consistently watering it to make the plant grow well and yield the desired fruits.

This made me advise the mothers to wish not only for healthy and intelligent children (as most of the mothers do) but also for children with good qualities. It was sheer joy to learn that Talking to the Baby children are well-behaved and stand apart as a cut above the rest. This inspired me to encourage mothers to use the technique to shape the baby for a lifetime. After observing the impact of the Talking to the Baby children in the family, I realized its wider implication on society.

Social Dimension

This book is primarily intended to help mothers get a healthy, intelligent and well-behaved child. The good news is that mothers can choose their thoughts and bring good human beings (intelligent and righteous citizens) on to this earth and contribute to making it a better and more peaceful place.

The need of the hour globally is to have more peace, as there is so much unrest in the world with increasing crime, violence, hatred, anger and jealousy among individuals. The only sure way by which universal peace can be restored is by changing human behaviour for good, which starts right in the womb. Like Frederick Douglass said, 'It is easier to build strong children than to repair broken men.'

Let's take a look at our glorious past. India, being a great country with an ancient civilization, has presented pioneers in various fields, such as spirituality (Adi Shankara and Swami Vivekananda), mathematics (Aryabhatta), astronomy (Varahamihira), economics and politics (Chanakya), medicine (Charaka and Sushrutha). Our freedom struggle and victory using mostly non-violent ways, set our nation apart as a shining star in the world arena. Great freedom fighters like Mahatma Gandhi, Subhas Chandra Bose, Bal Gangadhar Tilak, Sardar Patel, Jawaharlal Nehru and great kings such as Chatrapati Shivaji were all strongly influenced by their mothers.

In our culture, mothers, fathers and teachers play silent yet crucial roles in shaping the personality of the child and the three were, once, exalted to divine status. Tradition inculcated moral, ethical and spiritual values in the womb through the mother, later by the father and teacher and finally by society. Elders instilled moral values by repeatedly telling bedtime stories and proverbs. Our history reveals the evidence of tolerance, respect to elders and prevalence of peace in society despite poverty.

Because of rapid changes in social and cultural norms, we now see unrest in spite of prosperity in society. If the mother thinks and moulds the child of her choice by dreaming about the qualities of great personalities who walked on the earth before, she can write the fate of the nation in the womb. In the words of Alvin Price, 'Parents need to fill a bucket of self-esteem so high that the rest of the world can't make enough holes to drain it dry.'

I see a great future for our country and the planet when mothers desire and practise Talking to the Baby. Already mothers, who I have treated and who practised Talking to the Baby in the Womb are reaping the benefits of this technique. Our earnest endeavour is to see that this message reaches far and wide and our country shows the light to the rest of the world.

I have included an amazing array of feedback from ardent practitioners of Talking to the Baby stories of mothers, in their own words, to showcase how much this technique has helped them and helped shape their children.

I want to share with you the fact that my mother also practised Talking to the Baby in the Womb during pregnancy and she used to chant 'Rama Namam'. She gave birth to six children including me and all of us are happy and successful in our own fields. I am one of the living examples of the effectiveness of Talking to the Baby in the Womb.

Having come up to this point, I am sure you will be eager to know the concept of Talking to the baby in the womb and its amazing benefits. After discussing with many psychologists, philosophers and sociologists, I understood, it is the responsibility of all to spread it far and wide. The best time to know about Talking to the baby in the womb is before conceiving, but even if you begin your journey during pregnancy, it will greatly benefit you. I feel it would be easy for family and friends to pass on this wonderful gift to the expecting parents. Wishing you happy reading.

1

The Technique and Concept of Talking to the Baby in the Womb

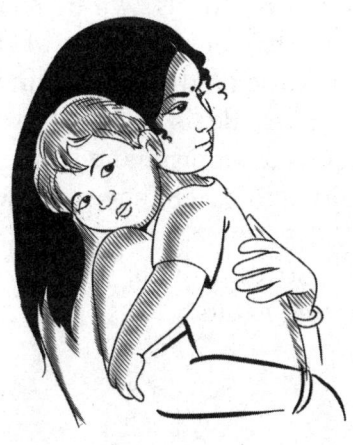

The more people have studied different methods of bringing up children, the more they have come to the conclusion that what good mothers and fathers instinctively feel like doing to their babies is the best after all.

—**Dr Benjamin Spock**

Sahana is Dr Andal's friend's daughter. She meets the doctor to have her doubts about pregnancy cleared. The narration is divided into four parts. Every part begins and ends with their conversation.

The first part deals with the emotional aspect: the concept and technique of Talking to the Baby in the Womb; hope, courage and confidence; how Talking to the baby in the womb helps the expectant mother face delivery confidently; and how to come out successfully with a healthy baby, even in the case of those who had a history of miscarriages; and the role of the husband in supporting his wife during pregnancy.

The second part deals with: mental aspects; intelligence and behavioural aspects of the baby; and the influence of music on the baby during pregnancy.

The third part deals with: physical aspects including physical dynamism and sporting aspects of the baby; vomiting in pregnancy; and meditation and yoga.

The fourth part deals with: sensory aspects; taste; and Healthy eating habits.

Doctor: Hello, Sahana dear, it's been long since we met. Your Mom said that I should spend some time with you; just give you a pep talk. You know, your mother and I have been friends since childhood. So I am glad you came for lunch. And congratulations to you, wonderful Mom!

Sahana: Thank you, aunty. I have lots of doubts—some silly ones, some serious—but ever since my pregnancy was confirmed, I have been confused. I suddenly feel so relaxed after meeting you. I'm sure all my anxiety will melt away now.

Doctor: My dear! Don't worry. For a prepared mother, pregnancy is a smooth journey and delivery is easy. Though pregnancy is a much-awaited event in one's life, the charm and joy of pregnancy are slowly getting clouded by anxiety and insecurity. The happiness can be restored by using a powerful technique. I'll narrate to you the story of a pregnant mother who was my guru in initiating this effective technique.

Sahana: Okay, aunty!

Doctor: Let's see Seema's story. It will help you understand better.

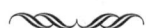

'You are already awake, Tara? Good morning! I am happy that you are an early riser.'

'See how beautiful the Sunrise is! The sky wears the most beautiful shades of crimson, pink, yellow and blue! Mother Nature is my favourite artist ever!'

'Look at those beautiful birds chirping, Tara.'

'Every form of life is so active as if it is its natural instinct.' 'Let's enjoy our cup of milk. You must be hungry.'

'Lukewarm milk is my way. Hey! Let's add nuts and dry fruits to it and make it tastier and nutritious.'

'I didn't know that you like it this much, Tara! Hereafter, we will have milk in more delicious ways.'

After some time

'Now it's time for some meditation and relaxation. Let's chant. AUM . . . AUM . . .'

'After lunch we'll have a nap and go to the hospital in the evening. We have our appointment with the doctor.'

Evening

'Come, let's go, Tara. Here everyone speaks Telugu—we will learn it soon!
   Chalo.'

On the street

'Madam, going out?'
'Yes, bhaiya.'
'Ah, it's good that he has come!'
  'I told you he is gentle in the way he drives his auto. I feel safe in it.'

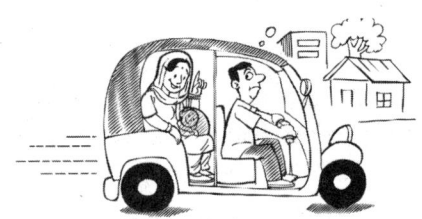

Always talking to her friend, but where is the cellphone?

'Madam, where shall we go now?'
'Bhaiya, we must go to hospital!'
The auto driver in his mind thinks to himself,
Madam is always on the phone . . . speaking to a friend . . . but I don't see any mobile phone in her

hand . . . maybe this is what they call some tooth . . . Aah! It's Bluetooth!

'We have arrived at the hospital, madam. Shall I wait?'

'No, bhaiya! It will take time . . . *mere paas apka mobile number hai* [I have your mobile number]. I will call you, then you come and pick us up.'

'Okay, madam.'

'Here is the auto fare, bhaiya. Thank you for the safe ride.'

'Thank you, madam! Bhaiya *boltihain mujhe* [You call me brother], I have the responsibility of a brother, right? You call my number, madam. I will come and take you back home.'

'Thank you, bhaiya! That's very nice of you!'

'Chalo Tara, let us go and meet our doctor now!'

'Tara, you are jumping at the very mention of the doctor's name! You feel so happy about meeting her every time. We must let her know how much happiness we get by meeting her.'

'Good evening, Doctor!'

'Seema Sharma! Good evening, dear! It is always a pleasure to see your cheerful face.'

After checking Seema, the doctor says, 'Everything is great with you. Every report shows good improvement and normality.'

'Thank you very much, Doctor! All this has been possible only with your guidance!'

'My pleasure, Seema. I've been wanting to ask you something peculiar I find about you.'

'Please go ahead, Doctor, you are a mother figure to me. You can ask me anything!'

'Seema, you are well into your sixth month of pregnancy. This is your first pregnancy. Normally, during pregnancy, women have issues such as vomiting and back pain. They feel insecure and get someone to accompany them to the doctor's clinic. But your attitude has pleasantly surprised me! I know your husband is a very busy executive, unable to be at your side always. Travelling alone in a town that speaks a different tongue is tough. Normally, all these stresses show up as physical symptoms. You don't have any complaints. How can you always be smiling and pleasant? How do you manage it all? Do you mind sharing with me the secret of your positivity and confidence, dear?'

'Oh, Doctor, I am happy because I am never alone! My baby is always with me! We do almost everything together. We cook, we shop and we are together always! We even meditate together. My baby falls asleep when I sing a lullaby.

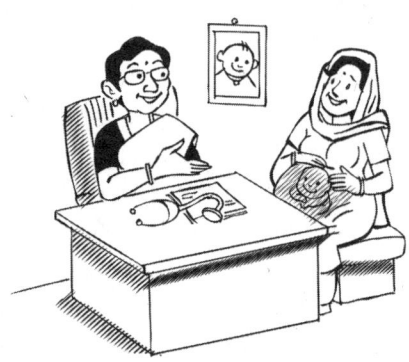

My baby is my best friend

And I must tell you this, although my husband doesn't spend much time with me, my baby gets along with my husband as well! They have their own time together, you know?'

'Oh! I didn't know that! Where's your baby now?'

'Right here, Doctor. In my tummy! I call the baby "Tara" to feel more connected.'

'Oh! That's amazing!'

'Doctor, whenever I talk silently or loudly, my baby responds with movements. We talk and we understand each other perfectly well! I enjoy my baby's company thoroughly. My baby keeps me happy and confident! My baby is my best friend and my caretaker these days! We take care of each other! Sometimes I talk to my baby loudly, unmindful of others' presence; many times others think I'm talking to some friend over the phone.'

'Eureka! The movement! So the movement is the language of the unborn baby. This is the master key to keeping the expecting mother happy and confident. I am so grateful to you, Seema!'

'Doctor, we are grateful to you! My baby loves visiting you along with me. It feels so happy and excited every time I mention your name. Today, I wanted to share this information with you, and you asked me just when I was about to tell you this myself.'

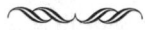

This was my introduction to Talking to the Baby in the Womb technique.

My mission has always been to make pregnancy an amazing experience for every woman. I want every pregnancy to result in successful delivery of a good child (healthy, happy, intelligent, with all good qualities = good child, for me). As I was struggling to find an effective method to make pregnant mothers happy and confident, I could see that Talking to the Baby in the Womb was the reason for Seema's happiness and confidence. Thus, the inspirational real-life experience of Seema laid the foundation of Talking to the Baby in the Womb. Mother talking to her baby in the womb is a natural and age-old practice. I don't think there's any mother who has not spoken a word to her baby during her pregnancy. But mothers think it's only a monologue, as the baby cannot talk back. They don't expect any reply from the baby. They are totally unaware of baby's feelings. When they are able to see the baby even before it is born, express their love, share their feelings and understand that their baby is there for them, its presence and companionship make them feel secure. Confidence and happiness will illuminate the way of expectant mothers—think, bond, relate, live, learn and grow along with the baby they carry.

How I Started Practising Talking to the baby in the Womb

It was the case study of Seema that inspired me to follow the 'Talking to the Baby in the Womb' technique to instil confidence and happiness in expectant mothers. When I explained the benefit of bonding with the baby during pregnancy and asked the mothers to talk to their babies, they used to give a quizzical look, smile and keep quiet; but I kept on telling them, because I'd seen Seema's experience. A year went by after I started recommending Talking to the Baby in the Womb; but the results were not encouraging. When I was about to lose hope, feedback from Sirisha emerged to strengthen my conviction. Sirisha talked to her unborn child and the baby responded, giving her a secure feeling and confidence during pregnancy. After birth, the baby responded to her words through his eyes. He was not a 'cry baby', and the kid grew up to be a happy boy, exactly as Sirisha wanted him to be.

How Does Talking to the Baby in the Womb Work?

Baby is connected to the mother through the umbilical cord, which has blood vessels. When the mother ingests food, it is converted into glucose (energy). Oxygen and glucose are carried to the baby for its growth and development through the umbilical cord. Along with the blood, the mother's emotions also pass to the baby. The mother's emotions trigger neurotransmitters/hormones that pass through the blood and trigger the same emotions in the baby.

For easy practice of Talking to the Baby in the Womb, I have divided it into three steps.

STEP 1

Every day, the mother listens to a particular song she likes and enjoys.

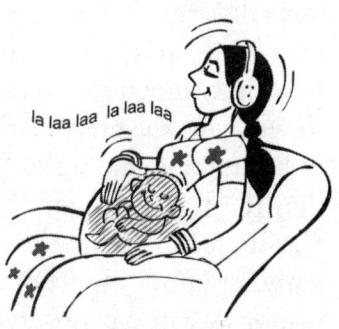

Talking to the Baby Step 1: Enjoying music

After a few days, she will notice that the baby moves whenever she listens to the song. Slowly, the mother will understand that this movement while listening is not a coincidence, but a regular definite response, indicating that the baby is also enjoying the song. The mother understands that the baby is capable of 1) listening and enjoying and 2) expressing its likes through specific responses of prompt, spontaneous and consistent movements.

STEP 2

Once the mother is sure that the baby is capable of understanding and responding to the song, she becomes confident that the baby will respond to her voice also. She talks to the baby by introducing herself, husband and her family members, and tells the baby how much she likes it and how everyone is eager to welcome the arrival. She wants the baby to respond to her talking and waits for the response; she observes that the baby, (sometimes) slowly, starts responding. She shares her activities with her baby and when the baby responds, the bond becomes stronger. Similar response can be observed on hearing the father's, older child's or grandparents' voice.

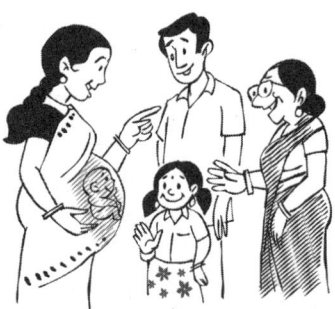

Talking to the Baby Step 2: Introducing the family

As more and more mothers started practising Talking to the Baby in the Womb, I observed other benefits. My initial observation was that it was a very good technique to reduce mother's anxiety and keep her happy and confident. The other important observation was that the baby's personality can be shaped through the soul-seeding aspect.

STEP 3

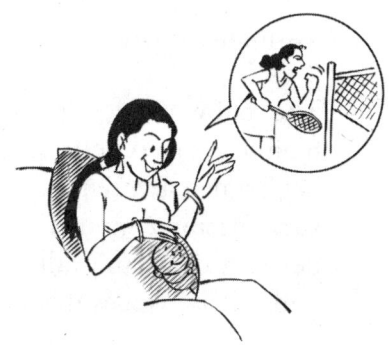

'Soul seeding': Once the mother–baby bond deepens, mother specifically talks about skills, achievements, and the qualities the baby should have and the dos and the don'ts. The result is amazing! The mother sees the exact replica of her mental picture in the baby.

Talking to the Baby Step 3: Visualizing the baby's personality and future

By practising this third step, soulseeding, personality is developed.

Benefits of Talking to the Baby in the Womb to the mother:

1. Makes the mother happy and confident, facilitating smooth sailing of pregnancy.
2. It also paves the way for normal delivery.

Benefits of 'Talking to the Baby in the Womb' to the baby:

1. It helps establish better and easier breastfeeding practice.
2. The womb song serves as a lullaby for the baby after birth.
3. 'Soul seeding' is a way of personality development and development of the skills of the baby in the womb. These babies talk early, communicate better, learn music and language easily and have higher IQ.

The baby inside the womb during pregnancy is a highly evolved self; though the size is small, it has heightened awareness and is extremely sensitive, as its subconscious mind is dominant. All the five senses are developed; it can't talk, but can respond to the mother and others' voices through its movements.

Why Do Certain Qualities That Start in the Womb Last till the Tomb?

The baby is directly connected to the mother by design—by structure (umbilical cord) and function. Feelings are passed through the umbilical cord. This is a unique period in human life where the baby lives under the skin of the mother, two lives are living in a single body.

The subconscious mind is dominant for the unborn baby and the analysing, conscious mind is silent during pregnancy; also the bond between the mother and the baby is one of love and joy. Hence, the recording (affirmation) in the subconscious mind is easily and effectively done by the mother and the impact of the recording is very powerful and long-lasting, like footprints on wet cement; this kind of recording to occur in the adult is difficult.

By twenty-eight weeks, all five senses are reasonably functional in the womb. Among them, hearing and touch are well developed. This has been proven in scientific studies. So, by touching the mother's abdomen and talking we can establish a strong bond with the baby.

The baby begins to hear and respond to sound as early as the sixteenth week. However, from the twenty-eighth week onwards, the baby's responses to sound are consistent and interactive. In his essay 'Ontogenesis of the Faculty of Listening', French otolaryngologist and inventor Alfred A. Tomatis wrote that the cutaneous sensory cells are analogous to Corti cells. Thus, the skin is full of receptors that respond to vibration, pressure and movement, and Tomatis viewed it as an extended auditory surface.* How amazing is that!

Dr Tomatis warns mothers that the earliest experiences of sound in the womb can have a stimulating or

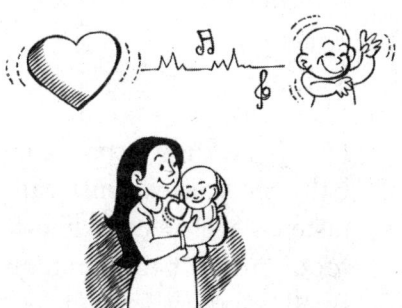

Mother's heartbeat is the womb music

---

* Tomatis, Alfred A. 'Ontogenesis of the Faculty of Listening', In T. R. Verny (Ed.), *Pre- and Peri-Natal Psychology: An Introduction* (New York: Human Sciences Press, 1987), pp. 23–35.

discouraging effect on the baby's desire to listen and communicate. If your voice is chronically shrill, angry and alarming, it is possible that your preborn will learn to become afraid of it. Try humming, singing, crooning and speaking softly. The foetus learns language and emotions through the mother's voice.

Hearing Heart Sounds and Connection

The mother's heartbeat is the sound the baby hears continuously. This is the non-stop background music in which the baby grows. This is why the baby strikes an immediate relationship with the mother. When the baby is born and starts crying, the mother holds it close to her chest and rests its head on her shoulder; it stops crying because it hears her heartbeat and feels safe and comfortable.

Taste

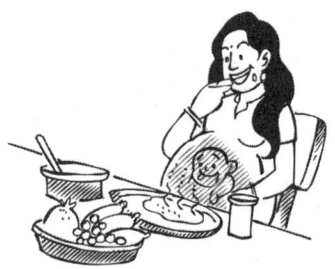

Both enjoying food

Do you know that the baby in your womb can taste as well as smell the food? Some babies retain smell memory and food preferences in the future. According to scientists Julie A. Mennella, and Gary K. Beauchamp, 'the fetus is exposed to flavours from the maternal diet in the amniotic fluid' and shows swallowing pattern changes depending on the flavour—evidence that the unborn child can 'taste' what the mother eats.*

Smell

Babies surpass adults in differentiating smells. Several years ago, Aiden Macfarlane conducted a test where he asked nursing mothers to wear gauze pads inside their bras between feedings. He placed a pad on either side of the infants' heads; the baby's own mother's pad on one side, and another mother's on the other side. Almost all the infants recognized their mother's pads by turning toward them.

Unbelievably accurate! According to Manella, 'It's possible that in the first few hours after birth, a baby's sense of smell may be more important in helping him identify his mother than his vision is'. By the age of one week, a baby can pick out her mother's voice from a group of other women's voices and, at two weeks, can recognize that the mother's voice and face belong together.†

Touch

The baby receives continual tactile and kinesthetic stimulation through touch in the womb, the movement of the mother, the amniotic fluid and the muscular

---

* Mennella, Julie A., and Beauchamp, Gary K. 'The Early Development of Human Flavor Preferences'. *American Journal of Clinical Nutrition*, Vol 65, no. 4 (1997).
† Verny, Thomas. *Pre-Parenting: Nurturing Your Child from Conception* (Simon & Schuster, 2003).

walls of the uterus and placenta. During pregnancy, the baby responds well through its movements if the mother's abdomen is gently stroked and she utters endearing words to the baby. It makes the baby feel secure. After birth, massage therapy helps in keeping babies awake and active. Newborns placed skin to skin with their mothers were calm and quiet.

Vision

A baby's eyes form early in pregnancy and continue to grow till the baby is two years old. The baby can perceive a bright light shining on the mother's abdomen; if the light is particularly bright, he will even lift his hands to shield his eyes.

Learning

'Our brains are primed for language in the womb', suggests deCasper's work. As a result of this natural programming, infants when they are four days old, can distinguish language from other sounds and begin to prefer not just their mother's voice but also their mother's language. The foetus undoubtedly experiences the mother's mental states, such as stress, relaxation, sleeping, walking, aerobic exercise, contentment and anger.

Maternal Stress

As in everything else, stress plays the spoilsport in the smooth and harmonious journey of pregnancy.

A study found a significant connection between prenatal stress and the outcome of a pregnancy, including low birth weight and premature birth.[*] Those with high levels of pregnancy anxiety (about baby and delivery process), were likely to go for premature birth. It is found that monetary and family problems resulted in low birth weight.

> **Fels Research:**
>
> Fels Research Institute, Ohio, did a study which demonstrated the way an unborn baby reacts to stress in its own way and this gave clues about the child's future personality. A loud noise was made near the mother and the fetal response was observed.
>
>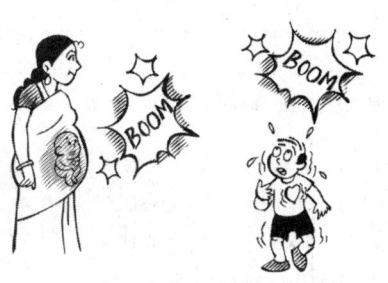
>
> Fels research: Startling response to loud music
>
> Two types of responses were noted.
>
> 1. **The low reactors:** There was steadiness of foetal heartbeat and the foetuses were less

---

[*] Wadhwa, Pathik D., Sandman, Curt A. 'The Association between Prenatal Stress and Infant Birth Weight and Gestational Age at Birth: A Prospective Investigation', *American Journal of Obstetrics and Gynecology*, Vol. 169, no. 4 (1993), pp. 858–65.

upset by the noise. Fifteen years later, these youngsters rarely got upset and were in control of their emotions and behaviour.
2. **Overreactors:** There were fluctuations in foetal heart rate.
   Fifteen years later they were highly emotional.

The impact of Talking to the Baby in the Womb on the babies is not always the same because it depends on the attitude of the mother. Broadly, there are two types of mothers: nurturing and managing mothers.

Nurturing Mother

She perceives the baby as part of her own self. She knows that the baby is capable of feeling and communicates easily and effectively. She cherishes Talking to the Baby in the Womb, includes and involves it in her day-to-day activities.

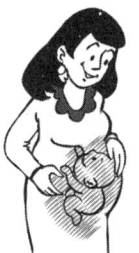 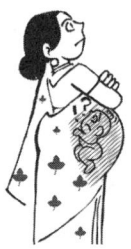

Nurturer: Mother lovingly touches baby's hand

Manager: You should become a genius, she commands

The baby enjoys her company, feels secure and responds through smooth and harmonious movements, she lovingly adapts to the baby and thoroughly enjoys its company. Thus a strong bond develops between the mother and the baby through Talking to the Baby in the Womb. As the mother talks to the baby loudly (or silently in her mind), she understands its likes and dislikes through its response (movement). Verily, the baby in the womb becomes (in some cases) a family member even before it is born.

When the bond strengthens, being (personality) is strengthened. Being refers to the inner self of the person—the personality, the finer qualities that define them, such as love, generosity, hope, faith, patience, perseverance. Having (ability or achievement) refers to the skills, abilities, knowledge and achievements. Having has a limited bandwidth. When being is added to it, the bandwidth becomes unlimited.

> *Nurturing mom = strong bonding + affirmation with love and care + belief = extraordinary and long-lasting results (personality + achievement and Skills)*
> *Managing mom = Weak bonding + affirmation mechanical + belief (only achievement) (only skills) = Expected results*

Incredible Effect of Personality with Skills

When Talking to the Baby in the Womb is done with love and care and strong bonding is created, the baby's personality is strengthened. The baby is happy and secure, and comes in total alignment with the mother. When it is in alignment with the mother's feelings, it is able to perceive the mother's desire and determines to fulfil and achieve it. When the mother expresses her desire (Talking to the Baby in the Womb), the baby responds through movements and reassures the mother. The mother becomes confident about the outcome. There is no stress for mother or the baby. The baby achieves short-term and long-term desires of the mother, easily and effortlessly, at the appropriate time. It's like a masterpiece sculpture, artwork par excellence or music that touches the heart. The effect is amazing and incredible. The saying goes, 'When love and skill work together, expect a miracle'.

To understand the mechanism of emotional alignment of the baby with mother, let us look at the real-life example of music director Ilaiyaraaja, who is one of those unique composers, who could identify a single violinist making a minor change in the notes from a group of 100-plus instrumentalists. This, he said was possible because he was in complete alignment with the feeling of all the people in the troupe. This is how an unborn baby produces the magical effect, by becoming totally aligned with the mother's feelings and fulfilling her wishes.

Managing Mothers

They perceive the baby as a separate entity, a foreign body growing inside the womb. Some strongly believe that baby is inert and doesn't know and can't feel anything. They carry their babies more as luggage and hence feel the stress and strain of it and keep expecting the time of unburdening, which is the delivery. Some expect their babies to adapt to them. Some women, when they become pregnant, might think of their babies as if they were 'just lives' growing in their wombs, taking nourishment out of what they eat. These are the mothers who could send a message to their babies that they are not welcome. These babies could then grow up to be shy introverts who think of themselves as a burden to Mother Earth. They neither enjoy the company nor carry out the affirmation (Talking to the Baby in the Womb) with involvement. The mothers want the babies to achieve the targets and expect them to feel responsible and produce the results. Sometimes the babies also feel the stress. Hence, their excellence is limited.

When skills are focused more, sometimes communication is mechanical or stressful (bonding is not strong). The result is there, but it is like beauty without life, food without nutrition, music without meaning, success without happiness. It appeals to the senses, not to the soul. Every mother, irrespective of the species, has a nurturing instinct. However, it is dormant in the case of a managing mother. With proper motivation and practice, a managing mother can become a nurturing mother.

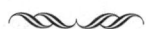

Now let us understand the meaning of desire, belief, affirmation, etc. Desire is from the conscious mind and belief is from the subconscious mind. Desire is the feeling of wanting something wholeheartedly. It gives the needed drive to do the affirmation. Affirmation is the process of recording (Talking to the Baby in the Womb). Belief is the feeling of certainty that it will happen. Belief is like a recorded song on a disc (belief = song recorded in the subconscious mind, disc = subconscious mind). When it is played, the same song is heard. The thought recorded in the subconscious mind as belief is translated into action by the conscious mind. Belief is necessary to translate the thinking into action, i.e. desired result (It is just like, what you sow is what you reap. Seed=thought (belief), plant=result). When there is lack of belief, in spite of affirmations, the song will not be recorded. We can't hear the song at all. That is why we won't get the desired results. So, belief is essential in getting the desired results.

There are three types of desires

1. **A weak desire:** When the desire is weak, the slightest doubt will shatter it completely. It is like a small lamp kept in the open air. Even a breeze can blow it out.
2. **A moderate desire:** It is like the flame of a gas stove that can withstand the blow of a breeze to a certain extent and helps in finishing cooking.
3. **A burning desire:** It overcomes the negative belief and puts in maximum effort to achieve positive result, overcoming obstacles. This desire is like a forest fire.

Affirmation or Talking to the Baby in the Womb is the process of recording. When affirmation is done with love or joy (strong bonding), it makes the recording smooth and perfect. The song is mellifluous and enjoyable to both the soul and the ears; it yields the desired results, which will be high-quality and long-lasting. Only nurturing mothers are capable of doing this. When recording is done mechanically, there is a certain type of friction; the desired results are obtained, but there is nothing extraordinary. The song is heard, reaches the ears, but does not touch the soul. Sometimes the effect may be temporary (achievement and skills). This is the way of managing moms.

Desire + belief = positive result.
Desire + no belief (doubt/negative belief) = no result at all.

- Desire + belief + recording with love (both mother and baby enjoy the process) = positive; these are the results that are amazing, more than expected and long-lasting, like an impression on wet cement. Nurturing mothers practise this; hence no stress to mother and baby.
- Desire + belief + mechanical recording (sometimes stress for mother and baby) = positive; these results touch the senses but do not appeal to the soul. This is the way of the managing mother.

Conscious and Subconscious Mind

Constituting 90 per cent of the total brain, our subconscious mind is our faithful, unquestioning and loyal servant. Its only function is to do exactly what we tell it to do (for better or for worse). The subconscious mind is just like a machine; it records, pushes a button and plays back. It is without direct interaction with the external world. The deep programme in the subconscious mind is running life like a tape, continuously repeating itself in a feedback loop, it keeps us stuck in the same pattern. It is on duty

24/7 and never sleeps. The subconscious mind doesn't know the difference between what is real and what is imagined, what is right and wrong. It is not creative.

We must remember that we are like an entity in the conscious mind, which constitutes the remaining 10 per cent of our brain. Think of our conscious mind as a 'gardener', and the subconscious mind as the 'garden'. Our *conscious* mind is tasked with interacting in the physical world and is responsible for identifying information through the five senses and making decisions based on what is relevant to us.

All of us got programmed even before we were born, in the womb. The responses from much of our preverbal programming dictate the course of our life until we become conscious of them and reprogramme or completely dissolve them. If people want to know what their programmes are, what in our life comes easily to us, it is there because we already have programmes to support that. If we have to struggle to get something, it is because there is no programme to support that.

So, the two minds learn differently. The conscious mind is called creative and can learn by reading a self-help book or going to a lecture, watching a video or reading an article. The subconscious mind is a habit mind. It is resistant to change. But we can reprogramme the subconscious mind. First, it is about recognizing the patterns with the help of the conscious mind. We need to question the facts, find out the benefits and disadvantages of the recording or programming. Then erase the unnecessary, self-destroying negative beliefs and reprogramme with appropriate positive beliefs. With repeated affirmations and visualizations with strong intention, the new belief gets strengthened and yields the result. So it is about habituation. Erasing old beliefs and reprogramming with new beliefs is like weeding out old, withering plants and planting new saplings. To do this is to literally rewrite one's life, its flow and destiny. We become reborn by deleting old programming that held us captive, captive precisely because we have forgotten about it, as it happened when we were in the womb before we had the thoughts and feelings we now have.

Now let us go through the amazing thought of the distinguished Bulgarian philosopher and spiritual master, Omraam Mikhael Aivanhov (1900–86). This is in consonance with our Talking to the Baby in the Womb technique.

> Throughout the nine months of pregnancy a woman not only forms the physical body of her child but, without realizing it, she influences the seed provided by the father by giving it conditions that will either help or hinder the development of its various qualities and characteristics. You may wonder how she does this. She too has to keep a watch over her thoughts and feelings and the kind of life she leads. Mother's thoughts pass through blood stream and reach the baby in the womb. This is what I call spiritual gold-plating or galvanoplasty. If the mother has lofty thoughts and feelings the baby will be healthy, beautiful both physically and in character and capable of overcoming all difficulties and diseases and all evil influences.[*]

---

[*] Aivanhov, Omraam Mikhael. *Education Begins before Birth* (Vij Books, 2011), p. 21.

He adds,

> The seed implanted in her womb may be of very exceptional quality, but if she has 'leaden' thoughts in her head (symbolically speaking), she need not be surprised if, later on, her child is cast in lead, that is, is vicious, pessimistic or sickly. Most mothers have no inkling of the tremendous influence their inner state has on the child in their womb. Later, after it is born, they begin to take care of it and look for people to educate and instruct it and so on. But by then it is too late. Once a child is born the dye has already been cast.[*]

Vikram Chopra says, 'Your thoughts and words are literally made into flesh. Every experience has an impact on baby's biology. Baby's solution is to consciously choose your experiences'.

Doctor: Sahana, I think you have now understood how a mother plays a crucial role during pregnancy in nurturing the unborn baby—a fact backed up by evidence-based studies. We'll now see examples from our ancient puranas.
Sahana: Okay, aunty.

---

[*] Ibid, pp. 24–25.

The Story of Parikshith

King Parikshit was the posthumous son of Abhimanyu and the grandson of Arjuna. To preclude the Pandavas' future generations, Ashvatthama decides to kill the child that Abhimanyu's widow Uttara was carrying at that time. He directs his Brahmastra at Uttara's womb. Terrified by the oncoming weapon, which would destroy her unborn child, she runs to Lord Krishna and takes refuge at his feet and begs him to protect the child in her womb. The Lord is moved by Uttara's faith in him and he immediately enters her womb and protects the child. The Brahmaastra salutes the Lord and returns without harming the child.

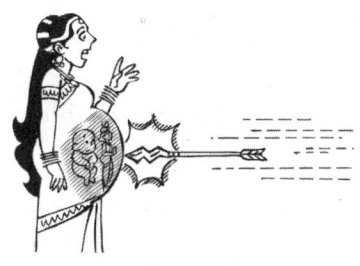

Lord Krishna protecting the baby in the womb

After birth, the child remembers the face of the Lord who had protected him when he was in his mother's womb and intensely desires to see that face again. So, when people came to see him, the child scrutinizes all the faces, hoping to catch a glimpse of the Lord's face. This is how the child earned the name Parikshit (one who

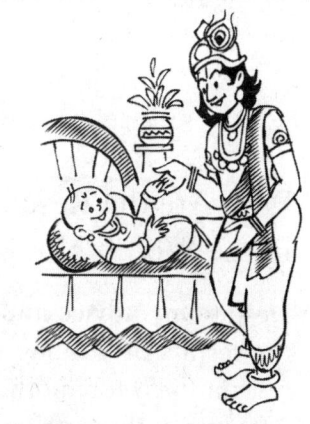

Parikshith recognizing his saviour, Lord Krishna

examined), and became famous by that name. You can say that labour is the perfect blind date, where at the end, you will meet the love of your life.

The Pandavas crowned Parikshit as the King and he was impeccable and righteous; all his subjects loved him.

Sahana: Aunty, I now understand the concept of Talking to the Baby in the Womb. After hearing about Seema Sharma, I am feeling very relieved. I'll definitely try to befriend my baby and, like Seema, become happy and relaxed. Are the results similar for all those who practice this technique?

Doctor: That's an important question, Sahana. We now know Talking to the Baby in the Womb works well, but the results for all those who practise it are not similar, as a lot depends on the intensity of the mother's desire.

Why Are the Results of Talking to the Baby in the Womb Not Uniform for All Mothers?

Despite my advice and continuous follow-up, I found the results of Talking to the Baby in the Womb were not uniform for mothers from different walks of life. After close observation, I concluded that when it comes to practising Talking to the Baby in the Womb, there are four types of mothers.

1. **Window shoppers**: These mothers take a look at Talking to the Baby in the Womb, just for information and never really make an attempt to explore its benefits. It is akin to taking a look at the menu card and leaving the hotel without ordering anything.
2. **Patient parrots**: These mothers spend time exploring the menu card thoroughly and have the patience to order and enjoy the item they love. They use this technique for specific benefits such as smooth delivery and healthy baby. They are happy with the expected results.
3. **Ardent Achievers**: These people don't just stop with ordering and enjoying the food they love; they study the ingredients, create their own recipe and cook new dishes *every day* at home. They have the patience and perseverance and intend to achieve more. These mothers make the best use of Talking to the Baby in the Womb, and get outstanding results for themselves and the baby. They develop a strong bond with the baby by sharing everything with it, almost treating it as a family member, *even* before it is born. Sometimes, other members of the family, such as the father and grandmother, can also talk to the baby. The mother observes the likes and dislikes of the baby she is carrying. She feels that the baby understands and cooperates with her. This gives her confidence and a secure feeling, and

she therefore does not depend on others for moral support, nor does she feel upset by hearing stories of a negative outcome. Delivery is a happy event of meeting her dear one. The baby grows up into a smart individual with extraordinary skills and qualities as desired by its mother.
4. **Fear savers:** Having gone through repeated abortions or miscarriages and conception issues, these mothers use this technique to come out of fear, achieve hassle-free pregnancy and a successful outcome. They ask the baby to support them and be in the womb till the ninth month. The baby responds through movements, and she feels secure and confident.

As the intent and approach vary with different types of mothers, so do the results of Talking to the Baby in the Womb. But it should be remembered that this technique has phenomenal potential.'

Sahana: Thanks, aunty, for the elaborate explanation. I'll surely try to become an ardent achiever. But this fear about delivery and labour grips me now and then. Actually, it has been there in my mind for a long time.

Doctor: Don't worry, Sahana! You are not alone. Every pregnant woman goes through this phase. Pregnancy is a period when even the most daring woman becomes timid. Let me narrate stories of some pregnant mothers who have shown extraordinary courage and confidence during pregnancy and delivery.

Sahana: Please share, aunty! I am very eager to know.

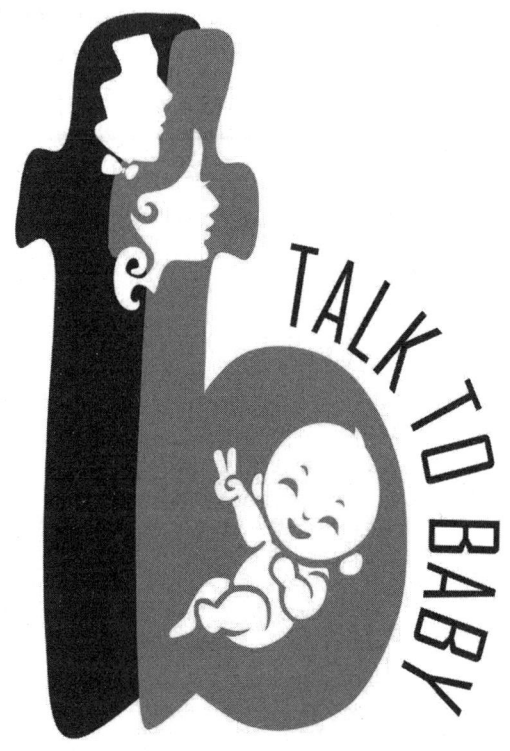

The Joy of two becoming three.
The love and hope of the parents are passed
on to the baby.
The baby is the gift of love to the family and society.
The greatest achievement of the parents is enriching
the resource pool of the nation.
Talking to the Baby is an amazing tool to
empower the intention.

2

Hope, Courage and Confidence

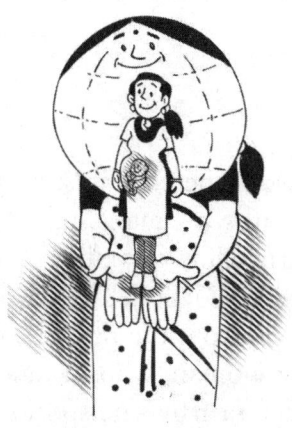

Some pregnant mothers are like grass, appears gentle and weak; yet powerful when faced with the storm. Some are like creepers gliding, bold and beautiful. Go forward in your boldness, beauty and contentedness. Trust your body to birth and know that the collective power of women worldwide will be with you.

—**Anonymous**

Doctor: Sahana! Let's see how Talking to the Baby in the Womb works wonders for the mother and the child. It helps mother establish a special bond with the baby in the womb itself; makes her confident in handling delivery and, later, the infant. The love and company of the baby gives her a secure feeling, courage and strong intention, which helps her overcome fear of vomiting, fear associated with miscarriage and premature labour and fear of labour pain. Outcomes are truly magical.

Sahana: Oh! Okay, Aunty. I am all ears. Please go ahead.

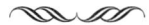

The anxious crowd gathered amidst the noise. A woman who was six months pregnant had fallen flat on the road in Bengaluru while travelling with her husband on his bike. The accident had occurred just behind their house. People from the nearby houses rushed to help the pregnant woman, whose name was Sreelekha. They took her to a nearby safe spot, made her sit and drink coffee. While her husband had fractured his hand and was in jitters, Sreelekha remained calm and spoke to her baby in her mind. She said, 'My dear baby, please be safe. It's all okay with you and me. I have to go to the doctor now just to make sure nothing is wrong with my body due to this accident. I feel all right. But I want to be assured of your safety now. Please speak to me and tell me that you are all right, with your movement. Please move and assure me of your well-being.' That very instant her baby moved, assuring its mother that it was safe. Sreelekha heaved a sigh of relief. For every mother, the topmost priority is the safety of her baby. But Sreelekha's position can best be understood if we travel back in time a bit and learn about the plight she used to be in.

Sreelekha used to be a very positive, bubbly and joyful daughter to her happy parents. She was bright and happy and liked to live a vibrant life. She got married when she was just about twenty-one and pursuing her MBA. She knew nothing about the nuances of relationships in her in-laws' house with new people. Even before she could adjust herself to the new environment, she found herself to pregnant. Her husband was busy, pursuing his career. Sreelekha felt lost and was not in the best frame of mind during her first pregnancy.

She had a thyroid problem (hypothyroidism) and was gaining weight. It was found that there was not enough fluid in her womb for the baby to be in good health. She underwent many tests and treatments to increase the amount of womb fluid but in vain. She delivered a baby girl in the eighth month of her pregnancy. But alas! She lost her baby on the third day after it was born. Sreelekha became more depressed and her weight increased from 75 kg to 90 kg, and there was no sign of any improvement in her health. Her husband realized that she needed better care and tried to comfort her in all possible ways.

They moved to Bengaluru from Hyderabad. Although a change of place helped somewhat, a lot was needed to console Sreelekha. She had been through several treatments and checkups in the meantime, and was told that there was a block in her left fallopian tube. Sreelekha was advised to undergo laparoscopy and the results showed that she had good chances of conceiving a baby with a clear right fallopian tube. Though she had been taking treatment, the feeling of failure, that is the loss of her first baby, kept haunting her and weighed her down. The future was very bleak; she had lost hope of bearing another child. During Sankranti, she came to her mother-in-law's place and consulted Dr Andal. She attended the counselling meeting, which is held twice a month on Tuesdays. She became totally free from all doubts and negative beliefs and felt relieved and relaxed after a long time.

How could Sreelekha make a paradigm shift? She learnt valuable information about pregnancy. Conception consists of two aspects: physical and functional. Physical factors (egg, tubes, hormones and sperm) must be okay, and can be assessed by tests and corrected with treatment. When all these, egg, tube and sperm, function together, conception occurs. It is the creative fertility potential that has to be expressed so that conception can occur. It is an inherent, natural function. This is akin to curdling of milk, germination of seed, etc. it is a behind-the-curtain activity. We don't have any tests or treatment for this. It expresses on its own pace at the rate of 10–25 per cent per month. Its

Hope, Courage and Confidence 37

expression can be accelerated by positive thoughts and suppressed by negative thoughts or emotions. Emotions control the fertility potential just like volume control in the form of fine-tuning. So, happiness, faith and positive beliefs trigger happy hormones and facilitate conception and it occurs easily. Negative belief, anxiety, worry, depression trigger stress hormones and conception is delayed.

Sreelekha clearly understood her condition. She had conceived her first baby when she had not thought about it at all. Now her physical factors were fine. Only she was feeling worried about being able to conceive. This was what was causing the delay. If she stopped worrying, she would surely conceive again. This realization dispelled all her worries just as light removes darkness

Sreelekha felt so relaxed that she would not mind even if she did not conceive a second time in her life. In her own words: 'I felt like a newly married woman without a history of pregnancy. That one counselling session was the turning point of my life! I became so calm and positive.' Once during a gathering, an elderly person said that Sreelekha was a very nice and friendly girl, but it's just that she had not been blessed with a baby. Even at that moment, Sreelekha had not felt upset and had seemed hopeful of giving birth to another child that would bring all the happiness. She had not uttered a single word to counter the elderly person's sceptical remark. She was just feeling very optimistic and assured herself that next year she would deliver a healthy baby and prove all pessimists wrong. This attitude itself proved that her mindset had changed positively and that she no longer had any doubt about her becoming a mother again. She was happy and felt sure about her husband's care and hospital support.

While recalling those days with the doctors and staff of Dr Andal's hospital at Nellore, Sreelekha said with a heart full of love and gratitude the following words: 'The doctors and staff of Dr Andal's hospital treated me as a child. They suggested that I take vitamin tablets and I did, gulping them like they were chocolates. I drank aloe vera juice, ate sprouts and other natural diets without any thought of pregnancy.' Within two months of her mind becoming strong, her system received the treatment well and Sreelekha's pregnancy was confirmed. This time, she decided to take every possible care for herself and her baby. And, of course, her husband was determined to give his beloved wife the best care.

It was in the sixth month of her pregnancy that she had met with an accident. Had it been a woman with a weak mind, she might have unwittingly caused some damage to her baby. But now that Sreelekha had regained the strength of her heart and positivity under the guidance of Dr Andal, she had spoken to her baby, seeking assurance of its well-being through movement, and the baby readily obliged. Sreelekha started treating her baby as a new member of the family and introducing other members of the family to the baby in her womb. The baby understood her introductions perfectly and responded well.

Hope, Courage and Confidence

Till her eighth month, though she had been going to Bengaluru for check-ups, the doctors in Nellore had been giving her guidance regularly over the phone. Sreelekha came to Nellore in her eighth month and strongly felt that she should again be under the most loving care of Dr Andal, until she delivered her angel-like daughter. Baby Amrutha came as the greatest blessing to Sreelekha and her beloved family. When Amrutha was born, she had sharp nails. When she was just one week old, she would put her fingers into her mouth and scratch her face with her sharp nails. Sreelekha used to tell her baby Amrutha to take her fingers out of her mouth and keep them away from her face. So good was her understanding and rapport with her mother that Amrutha would obey her mother. Now, Amrutha understands people's messages from their facial expressions and tone of voice and responds accordingly, much to the surprise and delight of her loving family. The very happy and grateful Sreelekha says, 'Dr Andal's hospital is my temple! Ma'am helped me evolve from caterpillar to butterfly [metamorphosis].'

Sahana: Aunty, the story of Sreelekha is very inspiring. It shows us that even after a setback, we can rise and move on.

Why do expectant mothers in general feel anxious when good medical care and experienced doctors are available? In fact, they should feel more secure and safe.

*Doctor: Yes, Sahana. In the past, elders had good rapport with youngsters and were considered strong supporting pillars of the family. They nipped the anxiety in the bud and made expectant mothers feel secure. With their keen observation and reflection, they formed protocols in align*ment *with tradition and prepared expectant mothers physically and mentally. That was why pregnancy and delivery were peaceful despite the lack of medical knowledge and facilities in those days. Nowadays, in spite of the availability of information from Google, advanced technology for diagnosis and state-of-the-art treatment, there is a lacuna in the area of reassurance to expectant mothers. All the treatment given is only for the body. The anxiety and the fear are neither addressed by the medical fraternity nor by the family. Because of the change in the social structure, family expects doctors to give reassurance.*

Sahana, there are two common fears expectant mothers have: fear of labour pain and fear of miscarriage.

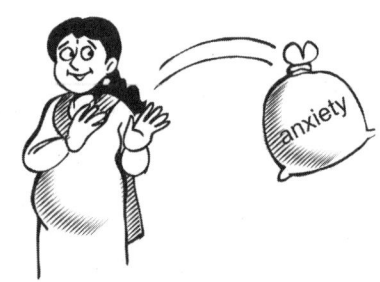

Removing anxiety hastens conception

Significant guidance comes from Dr Verny, who says,

> The normal well-adjusted woman who feels good about her pregnancy will make the transition to motherhood smooth as she makes every other critical transition in her life. If she is relaxed, confident, and looking forward to the birth of her child, chances are very good that her delivery will be simple and trouble-free. If she is rocked with doubts and worries and is in conflict about the prospect of becoming a mother, the risk of complications rises accordingly.*

Long-standing fear and anxiety result in physical effects both in mother and baby. They should be given knowledge, motivation and moral support.

Sahana: Aunty, why is there a tremendous increase in fear of labour pain these days?
Doctor: Yes, Sahana, you are right. Let's see the reasons for this.

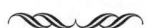

1) **Societal change:** The disappearance of the joint family system and the emergence of the nuclear family system has resulted in the lack of moral

---
* Verny with Kelly. *Secret Life*, p. 132.

support. Also, today's families are often separated by long distances, resulting in a sense of isolation.
2) **Stress:** Even in the past, there were dangers such as wars. But the pace of change today makes it different. Things are changing so rapidly that there is very little adjustment time.
3) **Visual exaggeration:** Movies depicting labour pain as unbearable make pregnant women believe that they wouldn't be able to cope with it.
4) **Lack of preparedness:** Elders expressing doubt that present-day mothers may not be able to endure labour pain as they are not used to strenuous household work. This can be an impediment to future mothers feeling confident in their abilities.
5) **Word-of-mouth campaign:** Some women may hear stories of other women's difficult labour and become affected by it. This could make them fearful of the delivery experience, heightening their anxiety and, possibly pain.

The Effects of Fear on the Mother

Fear can have many effects on the pregnancy: Pre-term labour, post-term pregnancy, small-for-gestational-age babies, precipitous labour, prolonged labour, increased pain in labour, increased incidence of foetal distress, increased use of medical interventions in labour, increased caesarean surgeries (both elective and non-elective), increased incidence of postpartum depression and other postpartum adjustment problems, and impaired maternal-infant bonding and attachment.

On the Baby

Studies show that mothers under extreme and constant stress are more likely to have babies who are premature, lower than average in weight, hyperactive, irritable and colicky.

Solutions

In Tribal Communities

In tribal villages, pregnant women join together and sing and spend time together. This gives them confidence that they are not alone. And gradually they overcome fear by

- Seeing a brave woman who becomes a role model
- Elders instilling confidence by reassuring.

Thus, the fear melts away, leaving the mother feeling relaxed.

In the Past

Despite the lack of medical facilities, our ancestors could make delivery easy at home. They did physical and mental preparation for normal delivery.

1. Physical preparation: Elders would repeatedly say that those who did household work had easy deliveries. So expectant mothers did household work.

2. Mental preparation

   - Acceptance of labour pain: Mothers should be aware and educate themselves about labour and the process of delivery by reading books and talking to their doctor. People around them should help normalize the process of delivery and all the emotions that come with it.
   - **Secure feeling:** Elders kept reassuring throughout pregnancy, during delivery and even after the birth of the baby.

In Modern Society

Mothers need to actively prepare for their pregnancy.

1. Physical activity and exercise
2. Mental preparation: Knowledge, motivation and secure feeling dispel fear and instil confidence.

Sahana: How do you prepare expectant mothers for delivery, aunty?

Doctor: Sahana, I strongly believe that delivery is a natural process and the mind has a major role to play. Depending on the state of mind, a mother can have a happy, easy, less painful normal delivery or difficult, prolonged and extremely painful delivery. The truth is, occurrence of both these types of deliveries is in her hands. It occurs according to her belief and mindset.

We, in our clinic, enlighten the expecting mother about the mechanism of easy and difficult delivery.

What makes delivery easy or difficult is the cervix, the mouth of the uterus (womb). when the mother is relaxed, happy, confident or feels secure, the cervix is soft, thin and short. The consistency can be compared to that of a rubber band. It opens easily with less pressure and therefore delivery is less painful. When the mother is anxious, haunted by doubts and negative beliefs that delivery pain will be unbearable, the cervix is unfavourable, like a bottleneck and firm like a ring. There will be more pressure and hence more pain. We prepare them physically and mentally. Physical preparation is doing simple household work, walking and breathing and other pelvic exercises. Mental preparation involves imparting knowledge and motivation, clearing doubts, dispelling fear and instilling confidence; another important activity is our staff giving moral support, which makes the mother feel comfortable.

We suggest pregnant mothers see pregnancy videos by Andal Fertility Channel on YouTube, which cover all the information and knowledge regarding pregnancy to equip mothers to go through pregnancy with confidence. Videos contain medical information, experiences of mothers who have delivered. After long years of experience, I understood that educating the mother and her family regarding pregnancy and delivery removes her doubts and makes the experience of pregnancy pleasant with a successful outcome of bringing a wonderful child on to the earth.

Knowledge

- Labour pain is a natural function of the uterus and the pain is not harmful unlike the pain in injury or disease.
- Fear-induced pain is unbearable and our medicines are not fear killers. Only knowledge and confidence can dispel the darkness of fear.

Motivation

- Our modern mothers do have pain-bearing capacity; they only need to know the benefit. That's why we see many ladies willingly endure the pain of threading their eyebrows, ear piercings, tattoos, high heels, tight clothes, etc.
- All mothers should know that the three real gifts they can give to the baby are: 1) enduring labour pains 2) breast feeding 3) womb song (to be continued after birth also).

Instilling Confidence

- We encourage mothers to open up, express their doubts, anxieties and worries and get them cleared. This gives them a sense of relief and confidence
- Husband, elders at home or friends must keep telling expectant mothers that she can have a

normal delivery and that she will always have their support.
- Mothers practising the Talking to the Baby in the Womb technique find it easy to say that their babies will cooperate for normal delivery.

With such preparation, understanding, and friendly nurses and doctors providing company to expectant mothers during labour, happy, easy and normal deliveries are increasing in our nursing home.

A Few Other Countries' Approach to Childbirth

The Netherlands

Except in high-risk cases, pregnant women in the Netherlands turn to midwives, not obstetricians. Couples have the option of a hospital birth, but most choose to stay home. In that case, the Kraampakket comes in handy. It's actually a home-delivery kit sent to every mother-to-be in Holland. Once a baby is born, insurance pays for at least one week of home-care visits called kraamhulp. A nurse visits the new mom each day to take care of everything, from caring for mom and the baby to cooking and cleaning.

Germany

Midwives are so respected that by law a midwife must be present at every birth, while a doctor is optional.

Japan

Japanese women usually deliver in modern hospitals with doctors, but many still consider an un-medicated birth. There is a belief among the Japanese that labour pains act as a kind of test that a woman must endure in preparation for the challenging role of motherhood. Japanese women are discouraged from screaming in pain during childbirth. Instead, they keep calm and push on.

Sahana: Wow! Aunty, I now understand your formula for happy, easy normal delivery.

Doctor: Good childbirth education is the accumulation of wisdom, confidence and trust in the woman's ability to give birth. An important element is giving her secure feeling at home and in hospital as well. One supporting person, uttering a supporting word repeatedly during pregnancy and delivery works like a small torchlight that shows the way for a few feet and helps cross a long dark street. It relaxes the mind and makes labour easy and safe.

Dr Dick-Read said, 'The anxiety state of mother can be replaced by a sense of well being through the receptive months of gestation without deep psychoanalysis but with intelligent and sympathetic education.'*

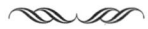

---

* Dick-Read, Grantly. *Childbirth without Fear: The Principles and Practice of Natural Childbirth* (Pinter and Martin, 2013), p. 57.

Let us see some real-life examples of the power of determination of a pregnant woman in overcoming the problem and delivering a healthy child. Here is the story of Yellavva, a twenty-two-year-old pregnant woman from a village in Karnataka, who showed extraordinary grit and determination in the face of adversity. In the ninth month of her pregnancy, she swam for ninety minutes through the flooded Krishna and reached the hospital. She took the decision to cross the river as there was no medical facility in her small village and the only way she could reach the hospital was by swimming all the way to the other side of the river, covering a distance of 1.5 km. She had not undergone any strength-training programme, nor had she been fed any special diet. She had never heard any motivational speeches either. But when she realized that her unborn baby could be in danger, she did not hesitate even for a moment to take the plunge into the choppy waters of the Krishna and swam her way to safety. The important point is that she had never swum before. Her brothers had tied dried pumpkins and bottle gourd on either side of her body to help her maintain buoyancy.

'This is my first baby and my love for it is enormous. I yearned to reach the nearest hospital in time. But as the water levels started rising menacingly and no boatman was ready to take me across, I got desperate and chose to swim as the baby is due to arrive any time. I took the hard decision as I did not want my baby to feel left out,' said Yellavva.

Twenty-two-year-old Yellavva's journey to move out of her flooded island village not only speaks of her grit and determination but her strong love for her unborn baby. No wonder she delivered a baby normally after two days. 'Being a mother is learning about strengths you did not know you had. And dealing with fears you did not know existed.

We will see another real-life example from our experience.

Swathy was a 'nurturing mom'. She practised 'Talking to the Baby in the Womb' very well and her baby was her constant companion. She did exercises religiously. When we told her that delivery is a natural process and labour pain is not harmful like other pains due to disease or injury, she analysed it and said, 'Yes, the delivery process is not difficult like rocket science. For ages, women have delivered without medical help. So, I need not worry about it. Moreover, I'm in safe hands. If it's mandatory for the baby I'm willing to undergo surgery.' Such physical and mental preparation resulted in easy and safe normal delivery for Swathy. Her joy knew no bounds when her baby boy opened his eyes and gave a big smile when she took him in her hands and called him 'Bujayee'.

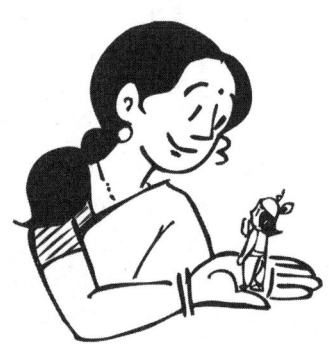

Jayashree gave herself confidence by keeping an idol of Vishnu in her hands

Pregnancy is a period where hormones are on the rise and so the expecting mother is prone to emotional upheavals. It is very common to see an otherwise strong woman crumble down under a minor setback or disappointment. In such a scenario, a miscarriage shatters her dream and undermines her confidence. She gets trapped in the vicious circle of anxiety, anticipating mishap and getting negative results. Here, treatment along with confidence alone can yield successful outcome of a healthy child.

We will see three real-life stories of mothers with past history of miscarriage and how they overcame anxiety, developed confidence and succeeded in begetting a good child. Jayasree was thirty-five years old with fourteen years of married life. She had had four miscarriages (one in the fifth month and three in the third month). She was obese and had hypothyroidism. She came to us in the second month of her pregnancy. She was very scared about the outcome. I told her we would take all precautions by way of tests and treatment. I explained that with the diet and treatment, 90 per cent success could be assured. If she was mentally strong and positive, 100 per cent success could be achieved. She thought over for some time and said, 'So 90 per cent is in your hands and 10 per cent is in my hands—right now, I am scared, but it's all clear to me. I will explore the ways to become confident.' Next time, she came smiling and showed me a small idol of Lord Vishnu that she was holding in her hand. She said she was keeping the idol in her hand throughout the day: This made her feel that God was with her and He would protect her baby.

Her pregnancy was very smooth and she delivered a healthy baby girl. On the third day after the delivery, when she wasn't secreting adequate milk for the baby, she prayed to Lord Vishnumurthy. 'Lord, you helped me have my baby; now help me feed my baby with adequate supply of milk.' Next day, her feeding was adequate! Faith and conviction trigger smooth hormone production, leading to sufficient milk production. I have seen some mothers taking medicines and diet to improve milk production in vain. Because their belief system was weak, they couldn't achieve positive results. The power of faith is magical! It works on the body and makes it work and surely potentiates the action of medicine.

According to Bruce Lipton, 'The power of mind can be more effective than the drugs we believe we need.'

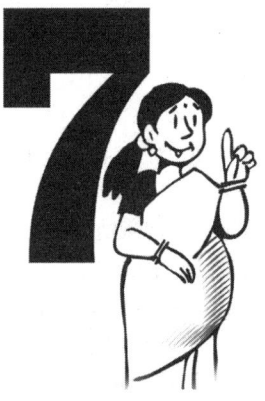

Keerthi was pregnant for the seventh time and came to me in the second month. She had had four second-month and two fifth-month and one seventh-month pregnancy losses. Her scan showed early pregnancy of five weeks. When I asked her, 'If it gets aborted, what will you do?' Without thinking she snapped, 'I will try till I get the child.' I developed an instantaneous respect for her patience and perseverance. No one had responded like that. Most of them would cry, some of them would say it was their fate; some would say they couldn't withstand

Even a seven-time failure couldn't dishearten Keerthi. She was determined to fight till success.

it anymore and would give up trying for a baby; a few of them would ask to be sent to higher medical centre in a city.

I realized that with this mindset, she would surely beget a child if she was made to feel secure. So I encouraged her and told her that we would be with her and give her all help needed to lead to 90 per cent success and 10 per cent she should cooperate, to which she readily agreed. I assured her that even if she aborted, we would try again. She felt relieved and happy. I would be with her till the birth of her baby. Keerthi came for check-ups frequently and expressed the slightest of doubts over the phone. I introduced her to our counsellor and all out-patient staff, and reassured her that all of us would take care of her. Slowly, she developed rapport with our team and felt the whole atmosphere was warm, friendly and secure; she felt happy that all of them knew her by name.

Her mother was ill and so there was no help from her parents. Her mother-in-law was supportive and did all the household work. Her husband was busy and many times she would come alone, as she knew everyone in the hospital and felt comfortable. We applied cervical stitch in the fourth month (to prevent miscarriage) and during admission, for two to three days, she came to know all the in-patient staff too. Her pregnancy was uneventful, except for minor complaints to which we attended very quickly, and made her feel comfortable and confident about the team. She was admitted two days prior to delivery and was relaxed. Even when she had pain, she was talking to all of us and delivered a baby boy very easily.

A few months later, she came and recalled her experiences. Before the birth of her son, she used to feel very shy and diffident to attend any social function. Even to wear a new sari she would hesitate. After delivery, everyone started looking up to her as a great role model and acknowledging her as a celebrity. Her mother-in-law was very proud that she had given her a grandson. Two years later, she delivered a baby girl.

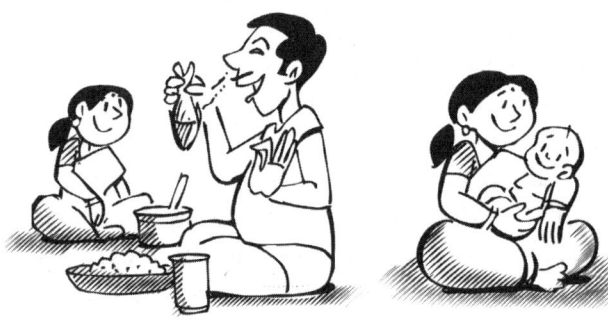

Selvi gained confidence on reflecting

What is the success mantra of Keerthi? Her intense desire was like a wildfire that could not be doused by failures. She was willing to face failure and continue till she achieved success. This determination banished all doubt, anxiety and worry. She gained confidence and a secure feeling due to the rapport she had developed with the hospital staff. Along with treatment, her positive attitude made the pregnancy a smooth sailing. The value of success after so many losses is very high. Perseverance surely has its rewards.

Selvi came from Hyderabad and had had three miscarriages at six weeks. Even IVF was suggested to her. Her eggs were not growing well. I told her to take a diet of mainly sprouts, fruits, vegetables and told her to do breathing exercise and yoga. I advised her to do it for three months and then we would do follicular study; her eggs would surely grow well, as the sprouts help in egg formation because sprouts are a good source of protein and vitamins. She appeared relieved. Two months later, she rang up to say that the pregnancy test was positive and that she was scared to go to the hospital. I congratulated her on conceiving. I told her to come down and that I would take care of her pregnancy. She delivered first a boy and then a girl. How could Selvi conceive so easily? When she was reminded about her achievement, she realized she had the capacity to achieve anything. She understood she need not go in search of ghee, as she already had butter in her hands!

Mother's Anxiety

Mother's anxiety is passed on to the baby. Scientist have observed the type of worry and the result in pregnant women.[*] They concluded:

- Anxiety and worry about pregnancy result in preterm delivery.

---

[*] Wadhwa, Pathik D., et al. Prenatal Stress and Infant Birth Weight', *American Journal of Obstetrics and Gynecology.*

- Life events stress such as financial problems, family and job-related stress result in low birth weight babies.

Research shows that as many as 10 per cent of pregnant women suffer from clinical depression, which can increase the risk of premature delivery or low birth weight. In addition, the intrauterine environment provided by a depressed or anxious woman may predispose her child to the same mood disorders. That means that therapy provided to pregnant women may also be 'therapy' for the foetus.

Deepak Chopra says, 'When you feel joyful, your body produces natural pleasure chemicals called endorphins and encephalins. When you are peaceful and relaxed, you release chemicals similar to prescription tranquillizers. Without stress, your baby's nervous system works smoothly. When you're calm and centred, your baby is able to grow peacefully.'[*]

In *Nurturing the Unborn Child*, Verny suggests exercises that a pregnant woman can perform throughout pregnancy. One of these is creative visualization. This form of mental imagery can programme one's subconscious thoughts, changing perceptions and responses from negative to positive. Verny writes, 'it has helped cure disease, enhance performance and improve state of mind. Used by ancient medicine men,

---

[*] Chopra, Deepak, Simon, David, and Abrams, Vicki. *Magical Beginnings, Enchanted Lives: A Holistic Guide to Pregnancy and Childbirth* (Harmony, 2005), p. 47.

shamans and yogis for millennia, visualization was the first line of defence against disease.'*

Bruce Lipton has even offered that a pregnant mother can affect her unborn child's genetic development. Whether it's called imagery, visualization, meditation or hypnosis, decades of research have established this process for generating a multitude of tangible changes in the mental, emotional and physical body. No matter what the situation, any parent can give their child a strong, healthy start. It begins with choices made during the pregnancy. The physical and emotional health of a foetus is shaped by the parents' environment and their emotional well-being. That's why it's vital to feed loving, positive energy to the foetus throughout the pregnancy. Doing so helps ensure a happy, healthy, confident child after delivery.

Chhatrapati Shivaji Maharaj

Jijabai was a very pious and intelligent woman with a great vision of an independent kingdom. When she was pregnant, she would pray in the temple of Jagadamba, the protector of the nation and dharma, 'Bless me with a son like Rama or daughter like Durga. O Mother of the Universe, give me some of your strength. Grant our lands independence. Grant that my wish be fulfilled, O Mother.' She yearned that her son may be part of a generation that could do this.

---

* Verny, *Nurturing the Unborn Child*.

Only a leader should be born who could unite the scattered, divided people.

She studied the intricate political problems of the country, in the company of experienced politicians and diplomats. She could see people falling into poverty in the once rich land and could see the culture that she loved so much being disintegrated due to invasion. She wanted to climb to the tops of forts on hills, to wield swords, to discuss political questions, to put on armour and ride on horseback during pregnancy.

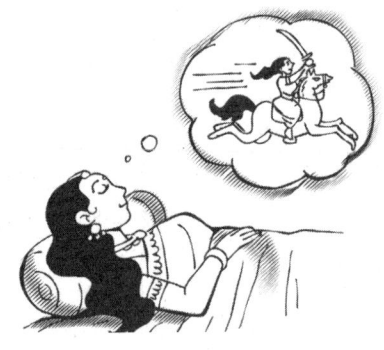

Jijabai dreaming during pregnancy

It has been said in ancient Hindu culture and is a proven fact today that the pregnant mother, by the environment she provides, by the thoughts she thinks and by what she wishes for her unborn child, does a tremendous effort to shape the child's life for good or bad. In the Vedic tradition, there is a series of sacraments and chants to be carried out so as to optimize the child's potential. Jijabai infused in Shivaji such a spirit, that was to emerge with great

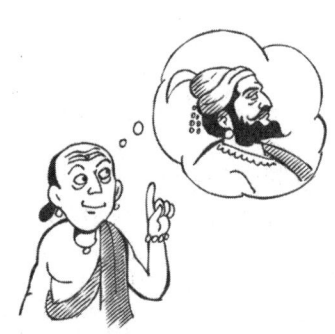

Shivaji Maharaj befitted the Chanakya's description of an ideal king.

force throughout his life. In Shivaji's impeccable, spotless character and courage, Jijabai's contribution is enormous. Jijabai is credited with raising Shivaji in a manner that led to his future greatness. When he was only 16, he captured his first fort Toma and that was the first step towards building the Maratha empire.

The ideal king described by Chanakya in Arthashastra is the one who laid emphasis on spying, who took full responsibility for all the results of an attack onto himself, who was disinterested in worldly and sexual pleasures and was well-versed in law and religion besides having an unblemished character and punishing subjects only when required. It may be said that Chanakya's dream king took birth in the form of Shivaji Maharaj after so many centuries.

Sahana: Thank you, Aunty. It is wonderful. After listening to you, I have a clear understanding that a mother can overcome the fear of labour pain. What's your formula for a happy, easy and normal delivery, aunty?

Doctor: Physical and mental preparation. Physical preparation by way of doing household work, and simple exercises like walking, breathing and sitting on the floor, butterfly exercise and squatting are enough. It's the confidence in the exercises that's more important. In my experience, I have seen many mothers who have doubt and anxiety, in spite of doing regular exercises, land up having a caesarean section. Those mothers who could do only household work, but were confident, had normal delivery. Another interesting thing I repeatedly observed is that some mothers, in spite of having fear of even injections, have had easy, normal deliveries; it's because they felt secure in the company of their husband, mother, baby or doctor and staff.

Sahana: Aunty, I understand exercises are important, but positive attitude is even more important for happy, easy, normal delivery.

Doctor: Yes, Sahana, you are absolutely right!

Sahana: I accept that happy delivery is in our hands. I'll slowly develop confidence to handle delivery easily. But it would be good if I could get some moral support from someone in my family. Better, if my husband spends time with me. But he is busy and is away frequently. Is there a way I can involve my husband during my pregnancy?

Doctor: I'm glad you have understood this, Sahana. Fathers play a very crucial role in the successful outcome of pregnancy. But many feel they have no role to play, and it is always the woman's job. Let's see some exemplary fathers. Please try to bring your husband along; it might benefit him.

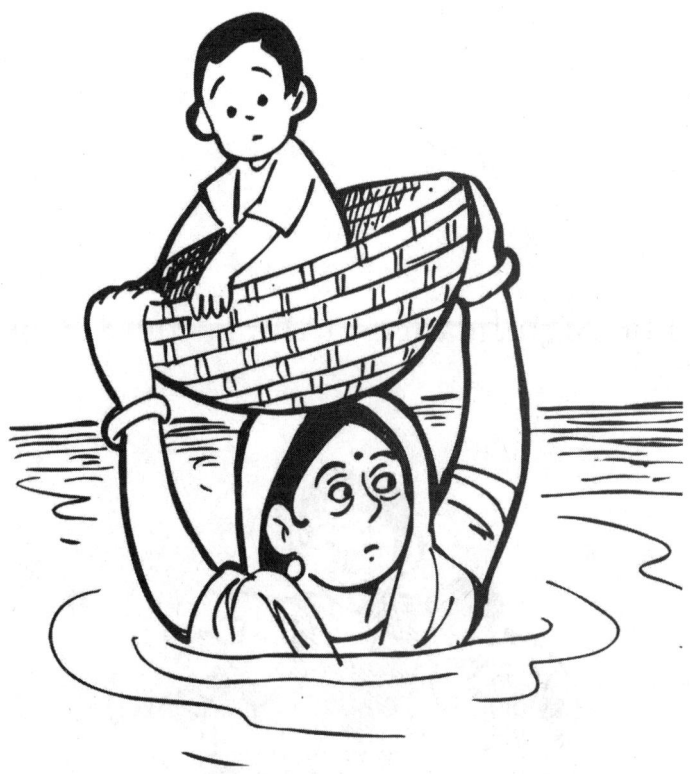

No language can express the power, beauty and heroism of a mother's love.

3

The Significance of the Father's Role

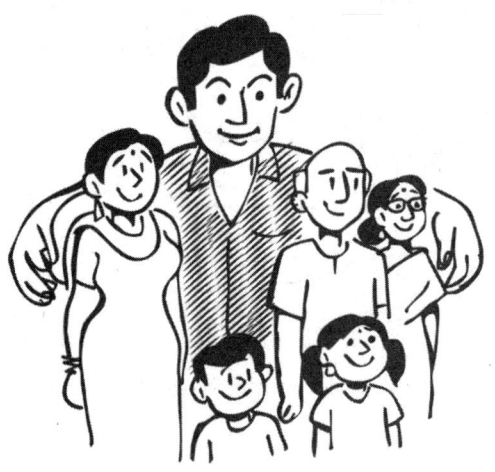

It's not flesh and blood alone; it's the heart that makes a father. The quality of a father can be seen in the goals that he sets not only for himself but also for his family.

—Reed B. Markham

Sahana: Hello, Aunty! This is my husband, Arjun. This is quite an unexpected trip, but the timing is perfect, as you said, this time you'll be talking about the role of husband.

Doctor: Hello, Arjun. Nice to see you.

Arjun: Same here, Aunty. I was excited when I heard about your technique from Sahana. I see changes in her. In the last few days, I found her to be more relaxed. It is amazing! In an effort to prepare myself for my journey to fatherhood, I started to google and discuss with my friends, and I got confused. When I saw Sahana change, I decided you would be my guide too. So, aunty, here I am, a naive father seeking clarity on certain issues so that I can support my family, I mean wife and child, and strike a balance between home life and professional life.

Doctor: Arjun, I'm touched by your sincerity. I am always delighted to see a caring and understanding spouse, because I feel the best gift one can give others is the feeling that they are understood, more so during pregnancy. Basically, husband's support gives the pregnant wife a secure feeling. In simple terms, it is like an anxious woman crossing a busy road in the company of a known person in a relaxed way.

Arjun: Sometimes I'm tied up with work for days together and that's when I feel off balance.

Sahana: Arjun, I am okay with it now, because I understand you'll always be just a phone call away. I think I can relax using the Talking to the Baby in the Womb technique; after listening to the story of Seema Sharma, I feel relaxed and confident.

Doctor: That's good. The role of a father during pregnancy is very crucial and can never be underestimated. Now, let's see some real-life examples.

Karthik: 'Krishika, come and sit. Today I am starting the autobiography of our beloved Mahatma Gandhiji.'

Krishika: 'Oh! So nice of you, dear! I appreciate your patience in enlightening and entertaining us with your reading. Baby and myself are enjoying these everyday sessions. I wanted to ask you where you got this idea from, Karthik?'

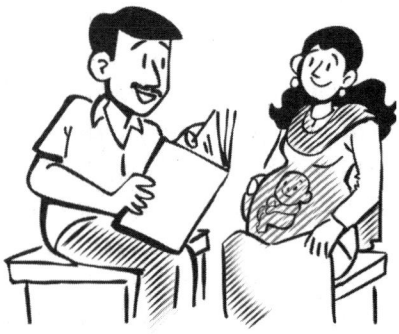

Kamala and her baby listening to scriptures read by her husband

Karthik: 'When I was young, my grandfather used to tell me moral stories.

I feel it had a great impact on shaping my personality. I thought my child should be better than me. I want him or her to be healthy, happy and intelligent, with all good qualities, such as good looking, strong in moral values, highly successful, and become a great inspiration to people. In short, I would like to see him or her not a mere person, but a great personality, a gift to the family and to society.'

Krishika: 'Oh, now I understand the intention behind your reading.'

Two years later, little Govind grows up to be an extremely endearing kid. He is always cheerful. His unique qualities the parents noticed are that he always likes to keep a book with him and unlike other kids, he is not interested in playing with toys. He likes his dad very much; puts on his dad's shoes and imitates how his dad prays before Sai Baba's photo before leaving for office. He doesn't trouble his mother. Once, when his mother was down with fever, he told her that he would take care of himself and not bother her. As a proud father, Karthik feels his son will surely become a good personality.

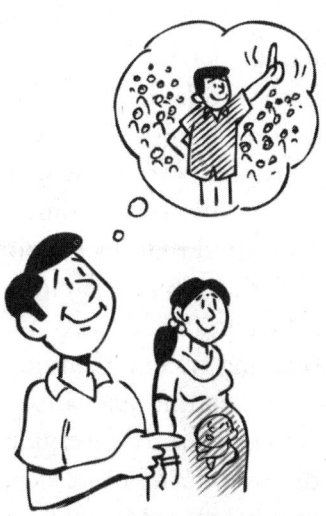

Father dreaming Govind will not just be a good person but a great personality: 'Shakhti not vyakthi'.

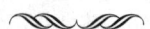

Pregnancy is a beautiful journey for every mother and father. Father is the central figure whose moral support means a lot to the expecting mother. When a mother is left alone to deal with it, the journey might seem tedious. He should be with her and the baby she lovingly carries in her womb. Just by his presence he can make it all beautiful and secure for both of them.

Dr Helmut Lukesch rates the quality of a pregnant woman's relationship with her spouse as only second to her attitude towards her motherhood as a determinant of the infant's well-being. Dr Thomas Verny writes, 'Virtually everyone who has studied the expectant father's role (sadly, so far, only a handful of researchers have) has found that his support is absolutely essential to her and, thus, to their child's well-being. A relationship with a loving and sensitive man provides a woman with an ongoing system of emotional support during pregnancy. And if, in our ignorance, we have disrupted this delicate system by rudely excluding the man, now that we have discovered, or more accurately, rediscovered just how important emotional security and nurturing are to a woman and to her unborn child, he can finally be restored to his rightful place in pregnancy.'[*]

Why a Father's Role Appears to Be Less Prominent?

As Dr Thomas Verny interestingly puts it, 'For obvious psychological reasons, a man is at something of a disadvantage here. The child is not an organic part of him.'[†]

The dynamics of a father's experience are different from those of a mother's. Normally, most mothers

---

[*] Verny with Kelly. *Secret Life*, p. 30.
[†] Ibid, p. 31.

feel more attached to the baby because of the physical and emotional attachment they go through during the baby's development in the womb. Pregnancy for a father is usually much more abstract. Fathers may not feel the need to get involved or worry about the baby until it's born. This approach can make the transition to fatherhood more difficult once the baby is born. Some fathers try to begin their transition into fatherhood during the pregnancy, but often they don't know where to begin. A father's frame of reference on how to attach is different from a mother's.

During the early part of pregnancy, he may feel life is normal with his regular routine still in place; this may continue throughout the pregnancy. Some fathers start to feel attachment to their baby when the mother starts 'showing' more, and the baby's movements can be seen on the mother's stomach. Others start getting involved when a name is chosen and they can start referring to the child by the name. Though the father may not be experiencing the daily 'kicks' and discomforts of pregnancy, involvement during this time is crucial in preparing for and attaching to the new baby.

How Important Is a Father's Role?

Every pregnant woman goes through emotional upheaval during pregnancy. She needs the support of her mother and husband. Being there for her and her baby and assuring love, respect and caring for them is of utmost importance.

What Can He Do?

Something as ordinary as talking is a good example: Foetuses respond to both maternal and paternal voices in utero, and hearing voices makes a big emotional difference to the foetus.

We have seen in cases where a man talked to his child in utero using short soothing words, the newborn was able to pick out their father's voice in a room even in the first hour or two of life. More than pick out, they responded to it emotionally. If they were crying, for instance, they would stop. That familiar, soothing sound tells they they are safe.

How Does the Baby Respond?

The baby's heart would stop racing, his respirations would calm down. This little newborn child would often strain to turn the head towards 'that voice', blinking through the bright lights, instinctively trying to 'see' the voice that it knew so well.

Balu and his wife Kavitha were excited to know about the Talking to the Baby in the Womb concept. They were discussing ways of putting it into practice. They used to talk to their baby in three different languages: Telugu, Hindi and English. They both started bonding with the baby and kept calling it 'Lucky'. The baby was reciprocating well. After delivery, the nurse handed over the baby boy to Balu's sister and she took him in her hands. Balu, as usual, called him 'Lucky Naana.' He immediately turned his head towards his father, much to the surprise of his aunt! Balu strongly feels that parents are the sculptors of the baby and the pregnancy period is surely the best time to shape this magnificent piece of sculpture. He also feels that if parents don't do it consciously, external factors will take the upper hand, making it an incomplete piece of art.

The Effect of Lack of Father's Support

On Baby

It has been observed that children of women whose husbands were away or did not show a keen interest in their progeny are either born prematurely or generally have low weight at birth.

On Mother

Many maternal complications such as anaemia, high blood pressure and more serious ailments were prevalent among women whose husbands were absent.

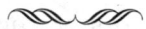

How Husband's Support Lifts the Spirits of the Mom and Helps in Easy Delivery

Malathi was coming to me frequently with complaints of loose motions and tightness of abdomen from the sixth month. I was worried that she might have a premature delivery. Luckily, she pulled through till the ninth month. Her father told me that her husband was in the army and so Malathi was concerned about his safety. In the ninth month, her husband Ashok came and told me that he would take care of her. He sent her parents home and stayed with her in the hospital, giving her physical and moral support. He made her do exercises, took her out for walks and stayed with her continuously. His presence gave her confidence and happiness. With her husband's support, she could deliver normally.

Asked about his concern, Ashok said, 'I found Malathi was tense and I wanted to remove her anxiety. I told her that delivery must be a very easy process. There are millions of people in our country, which means millions of deliveries have taken place. Hence it must be a simple, common and easy process. It's also a natural function of the body, so we need not worry about it. Malathi took care of me so well before pregnancy, for which I'm really grateful. And this is an opportunity for me to take care of her.'

The presence of a caring, loving and thoughtful husband who clears doubt, instils confidence and provides a secure atmosphere, turns obstacles into stepping stones. May the number of such nurturing fathers increase worldwide!

Fathers of the Past

Yesterday's fathers were expected to be good providers and taskmasters. They never took part in household chores. Emotional support was the elders' job. The expectation that today's father will be

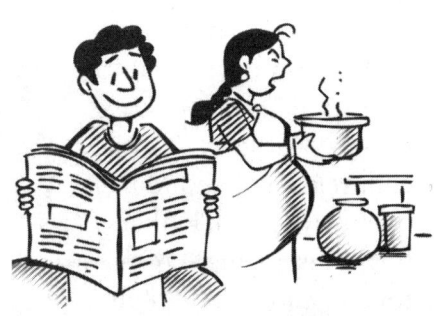

Father of the past

a sensitive caregiver to both his wife and children, calls for a difficult era of transition. In olden days, the joint family system served as a great emotional buffer, where elders took the responsibility to give moral support to the expecting mother. Cordial relationship existed among neighbours, who were like family members and offered help without expecting any favour in return. In sharp contrast, in present-day nuclear family systems, elders don't live with the couple. Sometimes we don't know who our neighbours are even after living close to them for decades. So, the burden of taking care of the pregnant woman falls on the shoulders of the spouse.

Present-Day Fathers

Many fathers have only nights and weekends to interact with their newborn. Added to this, the fact that more than half of all new mothers breastfeed limits dad's role as a source for feeding the baby.

Dr Ross Parke found that although men are slightly slower to warm to their children due to the fact that they are not as biologically or culturally primed as women are, now fathers and children are bonding openly for good. Fathers now kiss, hug, rock, touch and hold their newborn babies as much as their wives do. They are actively getting involved in household chores. A growing number of fathers have also started to take time off during the first few years of their babies' growth. Some fathers, though silent, their hearts are full of love. In some cases, the sensitive baby recognizes his unexpressed love and responds.

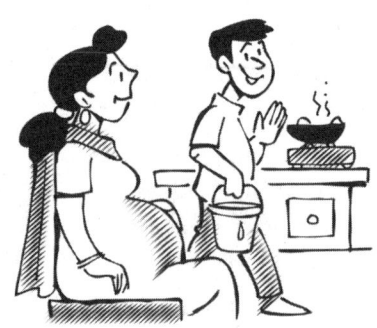

Present-day father reassuring the mother and helping with household chores

Balaji was a silent person. When his wife, Tulasi, was expecting her first kid, he'd come and just sit with her for some time. Tulasi noticed that as soon as he entered the room, the baby would start moving. She understood her baby was fond of

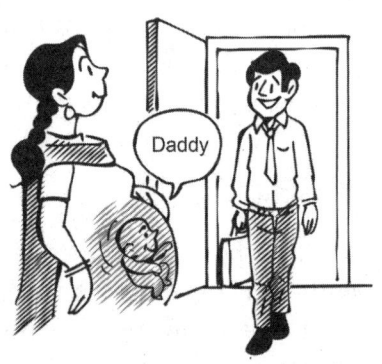

Baby moves when father enters the room

Dad, who was too shy to express his love verbally. When the baby was born, she looked into the eyes of her Dear Dad and held his hands. Now she is eight years old and she is still a daddy's doll.

Tips for More Involvement

Become Informed

Read up on pregnancy, childbirth and baby care. Talk to other fathers. The more informed you are, the more comfortable you'll feel. It's also good to develop a support system of fathers to call upon, should you need some help relating to your spouse during pregnancy or adjusting to changes after the baby comes.

Attend Prenatal Appointments

Expecting mothers feel happier when husbands accompany them to a doctor's clinic. When he discusses with the doctor about her progress and learns the precautions to be taken, she feels secure. Naturally, she looks forward to him staying with her during the delivery. It's a great way to show support for the partner. For the husband, hearing the heartbeat and seeing the ultrasound helps make the pregnancy feel more real, especially in the early months when the only outward signs may be a nauseated, tired and moody mother.

Feel for Kicks

A couple of weeks after the mother starts to feel the baby move, others too will be able to feel the kick if they put a hand on the mother's belly. Talk or sing to the baby—even in the womb, the baby can hear father's voice and react. Once the baby is born, he or she will be able to differentiate father's voice from mother's and others' voices.

Talking to the baby every day as a routine makes the baby feel continuously bonded with the father. The baby identifies the voice, touch and feel of father in the room or over the phone. What an honour for the father to be sensed by his baby in the mother's womb! By the time the baby comes, it will have befriended you. So the baby looks forward to its time to be with you on a daily basis. Have a particular time schedule every day, during which you talk to your baby. This commitment to your baby is one of the best gifts you can give to it.

Sendhil and his wife Radha are both employees. After learning about the technique of Talking to the Baby in the Womb, they became nurturing parents. Radha had stage fright and so she dreamed her baby to have excellent oratory skills, backed up by good memory. Her daughter has extraordinary memory and started giving performances

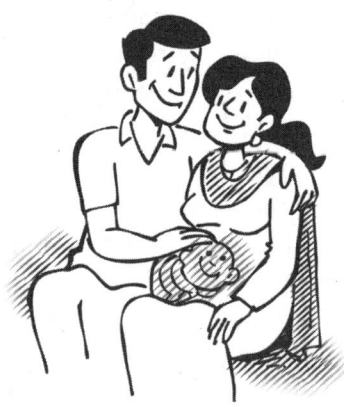

Present-day father talking to both mom and baby

at the age of three. Sendhil talked endearingly to the baby and bonded well during pregnancy. As she dreamt, he produced a stable and happy family. His vision of 'Prema Bharat' can be attained if all parents follow his footsteps.

Ramya and Vidhyadhar are a very understanding and affectionate couple Vidhyadhar used to take good care of her during pregnancy. He'd help her with household chores, asked how she felt and gave her medicines himself. He told her every day that he loved her and the baby very much. Every night his routine was to narrate to Ramya the whole day's proceedings in his office. He adored his boss very much and did his job wholeheartedly. One week after the delivery, when the boss came home to see his son, the baby gestured a Namaskaram by folding both hands, as a mark of respect.

Such is the sensitivity and understanding of a baby in the womb; such gestures from the newborn are amazing and incredible, but true! This result is due to influence of nurturing parents. When a mother talks to the baby with love and care, a strong bonding between the two is

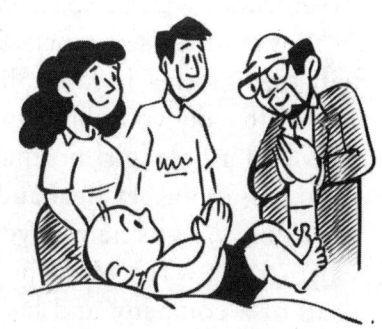

Baby doing namaskar to boss

created. This strengthens the baby's personality and it gets aligned with the mother, understands her feelings and is able to fulfil those desires easily. Such wonderful effects are possible only because of efforts of the nurturing mother. When the personality is strengthened, excellence is a natural offshoot.

In some cases, even when the father is far away, he is in regular contact with his wife on phone, giving her the most needed moral support. Sujatha was in her first pregnancy and came to Nellore to visit her parents-in-law. She was living in a far-off city with her husband Raj, who was a very busy executive. She came for a casual check-up and attended the antenatal class. Later she said she liked the hospital and would surely come for delivery. She was in regular phone contact with me, informing me about her test and treatment, etc. Though she had been telling me she would come for delivery, I never took it seriously, as her parents lived in Chennai, with a corporate hospital on the same street. Moreover, her parents-in-law were quite old.

I was surprised when Sujatha came for delivery with her mother-in-law. She said her parents would come after delivery. She was cool and composed and delivered a baby girl normally. After delivery, when I enquired about her husband, she said he would come after nine days as he was very busy. When I asked her whether she was missing him, she said that he was the head of a company and had a tight schedule. He had been calling her twice a day and talking to her and the baby. She felt very happy and secure with this gesture and was not missing him.

I felt great regard for her husband Raj when she revealed that he had stopped taking sweets after she was found to be a diabetic. This amazing power of husband–wife understanding was an eye-opener to me. Thus, the father can hold the protective umbrella over the mother and the baby by being bonded with them emotionally, even though he is physically far away.

Family and Friends

Grandparents and older children can also bond well with baby in the womb. When the whole family welcomes the baby, it is sheer joy for all. And the pregnancy is very smooth. After birth, the baby bonds well with everyone. The role of elders and friends can never be underestimated. They form a good shock-absorbing system by building rapport, making everyone open up, thereby easing the tension and anxiety.

Let me tell you two emotional and interesting incidents about the value of relationships. This is a conversation between a mother and her daughter. My mother used to ask me what the most important part of the body was. I would take a guess at what I thought was the most correct answer. Though I said 'ears, eyes, heart, etc., my mother wasn't convinced. She clarified, 'My dear, the most important body part is our shoulder.'

'Is it because it holds up our head?' I asked.

'No, it is because it can hold the head of a friend or a loved one when he or she cries. Everybody needs a shoulder to cry on sometimes in life, my dear. I only hope that you have enough love and friends that you will always have a shoulder to cry on when you need it.' Then I knew the most important body part is not a selfish one. It is made for others. It is sympathetic to the pain of others. People will forget what you said and did. But will never forget how you made them feel when they were sad, because what you said reaches the mind and how you said it reaches the heart.

One day, a person went to the market to buy grapes. The cost of a bunch of grapes was Rs 80 per kg and that of loose grapes, Rs 30 per kg. When the vendor was asked why this was so, he said, 'They are also good, but they have been separated from the bunch.' Similarly, when we are separated from our family, friends and relations, our value and strength also decrease.

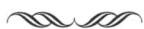

Deva Premal

Deva Premal is a musician known for her meditative spiritual new-age music, which combines ancient Buddhist and Sanskrit mantras, as well as chants in other languages, with atmospheric contemporary sounds. Premal met her partner in life and music, Miten, at the Osho Ashram in Pune (India) in 1990, where she was studying reflexology, shiatsu, craniosacral therapy and massage therapy. They have been touring together since 1992, offering concerts and chant workshops worldwide.

Best known for her top-selling chant CDs, Premal is a classically trained musician who grew up singing mantras in a German home permeated with eastern spirituality. Her albums have topped the new-age charts throughout the world since her first release. The *Essence* (1998) features the 'Gayatri Mantra'. Premal and Miten's record company, Prabhu Music, reports sales of over 900,000 albums.

Deva Premal began her journey with mantra in her mother's womb, as every day her father chanted the Gayatri Mantra—one of the most sacred mantras of the Sanatana Dharma. The mantra continued to be her bedtime lullaby after she was born. Many years later, she heard a friend singing the Gayatri Mantra and was inspired to put together an album highlighting its sacredness. Premal and Miten recorded *The Essence (1998)* in her mother's apartment in Germany, where she was born and where she had first heard the Gayatri Mantra.

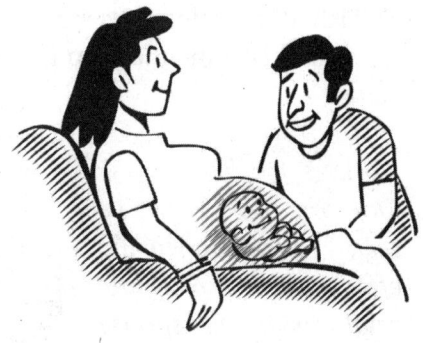

Father welcoming Deva with Gayathri Mantra before her arrival

Deva Premal brought this journey with the Gayatri Mantra full circle in July 2005, when she and Miten chanted it for her father as he lay dying, 'We kept singing for what must have been over half an hour, when suddenly the monitor showed that he was about to leave. I continued to sing, and the last sound he heard as he passed away was his beloved Gayatri Mantra. Finally, we ended with the mantra Om and the circle was complete. He had welcomed me onto this planet with the Gayatri, and I accompanied him out of this physical existence with it. What a blessing this was for me! It was the first time that I was present at a death, and to be at my father's, is a memory I will cherish all my life.'

A dad is someone who holds you when you cry.

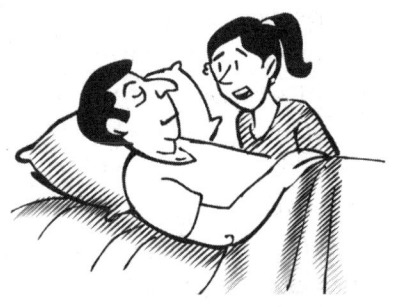

Deva giving farewell to Dad with Gayathri Mantra

Doctor: Dear, we've seen the nurturing effects of the root-like relationship of spouse and family. Roots support us during the storm to stay strong.'

Sahan: 'Aunty! Arjun and my mother-in-law are very supportive.

But sometimes I feel a little hesitant to convey my feelings to them.

Doctor: You should not have any hesitation or inhibition in expressing to your husband and mother-in-law what you want. For example, when you feel like sleeping due to fatigue and tiredness, you should frankly tell your mother-in-law. Imagining her reaction will be negative and therefore not telling her can result in the build-up of unnecessary negative emotions, manifesting as physical symptoms such as abdominal or back pain. This can be avoided. You should also take help from your husband, both physical and emotional, by telling him frankly what you expect from him and how he must give it. You must choose an appropriate time, when he is in a relaxed frame of mind, tell him your requirement. It should not be in a complaining tone.

Please understand that your husband and mother-in-law are not feeling the emotions or physical discomforts you are going through. Only when you explain and ask for help can they oblige. Often, misunderstanding arises because of lack of proper communication. So, don't feel guilty and hesitant to express your feelings. Be bold and ask what you want. Get the necessary physical and moral support from your husband and mother-in-law, especially during the pregnancy period.

Arjun: Thanks a lot, Aunty. The stories from your experience have cleared most of my doubts. I will express my love, concern and solidarity to Sahana and the baby. I will also share these insights with my mother so that Sahana will be more comfortable throughout pregnancy and delivery. In short, I understood mother's intention and father's support are vital for a successful outcome of pregnancy.'

Sahana: Aunty, I understood the tips about freely expressing feelings and taking help from others. The monkey is off my back and I feel absolutely relaxed. Arjun is very smart and intelligent and adores such people; I want this baby to be his replica in this aspect, so that he'll cherish this gift. Can I take some measures to improve the IQ of the baby during pregnancy itself?

Arjun: Wow, Sahana, that's very nice of you. I'm thrilled.

Doctor: Sahana, you can lay the blueprint of the baby during pregnancy for health, intelligence and behaviour. They can certainly be groomed during pregnancy. The seeds can be sown in pregnancy, so that just watering after birth will yield the desired result (personality and skills).

Doctor: Come, Sahana and Arjun. We'll take a short tea break and visit our small garden. Later, we'll see how to improve intelligence during pregnancy.

Arjun: Fine with us, aunty.

Dear Daddy,
I may find a prince some day,
but you will always be my king.

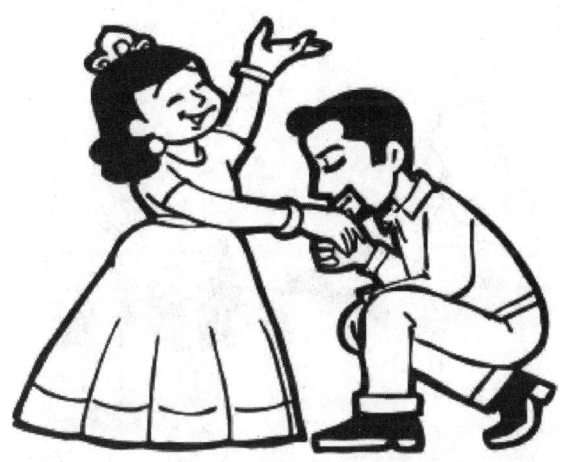

4

Intelligence

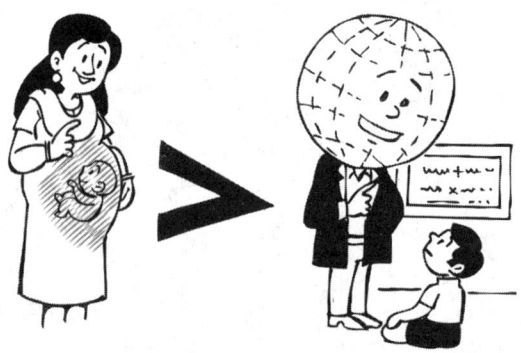

What a child learns in the womb cannot be learnt on the earth. Mother is the first guru of the child. Intelligence can be nurtured, developed and expanded to levels not yet imaginable, if we begin at the earliest stages of life, before birth.

—Akio Morita, one of the founders of Sony

Sahana: Aunty, is it possible to give birth to an intelligent baby using the Talking to the Baby technique?

Doctor: Yes, Sahana! It is absolutely possible to stimulate cognitive abilities of the baby during pregnancy. I can share a number of experiences. According to Vedic scriptures, the baby's mind is like fertile soil and has the potential to absorb everything. Parents can make use of this opportunity to make learning easy for the baby in the womb. David Chamberlain, the pioneer in prenatal and perinatal psychology, states that, 'The truth is, much of what we have traditionally believed about babies is false. They are not simple beings but complex and ageless—small creatures with unexpectedly large thoughts. *I'll tell you Meethu's story.*

Arjun: Aunty, I'm absolutely delighted to listen to stories about intelligence'

'Hello, Dr Andal and Dr Bhaskar! It's very nice to see you in a restaurant!'

'Hello, Manorama and Manisha! The "M" sisters! Nice to see you both. How is Meethu?'

'I delivered Meethu with your guidance. She is doing very well, both in life and in her studies. She is the topper in class tenth!'

---

* Chamberlain, David. *The Mind of Your Newborn Baby* (North Atlantic Books, 1998), xiii).

'Wow, that's wonderful news, Manorama! Years run by so fast! Remember, you had come to me for your second pregnancy, and I'd suggested to you Talking to the Baby in the Womb?'

'How can I forget that experience, Doctor. I started practising talking to my baby right from the second month of my pregnancy. Slowly, I observed that my baby understood all that I said to her, and she started responding through her movements. I used to tell Meethu during pregnancy to be as smart as my sister Manisha and Manisha, too, used to talk to her while I took naps.'

Manisha joins in, 'Yes, Doctor, I used to talk to Meethu a lot. And we noticed to our surprise when Meethu was just one-and-a-half to two years old, she used to learn many things without any of us teaching her,' Manisha said.

'Yes, Manisha, the human body is a form comprising of trillions of intelligent cells. Every human is a powerhouse of collective intelligence, and every life form is awesomely created. I feel no foetus should be thought of or treated as an inert being that some mothers carry the baby mechanically just like luggage.'

'You are absolutely right, Doctor, and you've said it very beautifully!'

'Meethu would sit with me when I was helping her elder brother with lessons and listen with great attention. She seemed to understand his lesson very easily. She always used to carry a notebook and pen and liked to write on her own. Doctor, when I took Meethu to school the first day, she was all inquisitive and all eyes and ears to know about everything that happened there. When we came across a board near the principal's office, Meethu made me stop and asked what it was.

I explained that it was toppers' list of class ten over the years. Without any hesitation, she told me in a confident tone that her name, too, would appear on it,' said Manorama.

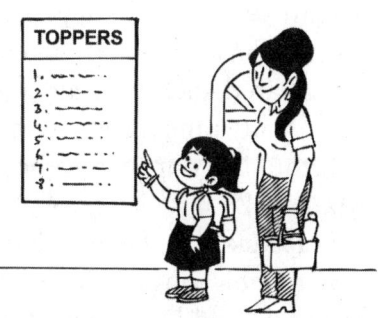

Meethu saying that her name will appear on the school toppers' list

'It is amazing to know and experience how a very small step taken by a pregnant woman can go a long way in giving the best life to a child!'

Manisha adds, 'Yes, doctor, and whenever Manorama was busy, I used to go to pick Meethu from her school in the evenings and many times I caught her staring at that board with interest. And today her name found its place on that same board.' All this is due to your 'Talking to the Baby in the Womb, Doctor.'

'Awesome Manisha, I am so happy that as per Manorama's wish, our little Meethu has blossomed to be as smart as you are!'

'I feel so humbled to listen to such words from you, Doctor.'

'No, Manisha, you are a very smart microbiologist and you are involved in breakthrough research that will be a boon to humanity!'

'Doctor, we are happy to remember your analogy of the clean board to write the first best words! Yes, the mother's womb is the clean board and parents write the first best lessons in the form of knowledge. We are seeing the living example of Meethu!'

Dr Bhaskar replies, 'I am so happy that we met you and shared such pleasant results of soul seeding! Oh, it's already time for us to start. Convey our blessings to Meethu and our love to both of you, Manorama and Manisha!'

'Thank you, Dr Bhaskar, we will surely give your love and blessings to Meethu, and we will bring her to meet you and Dr Andal soon.'

So, this is the story of Meethu, in which the intelligence was nurtured during pregnancy and beyond.

Human beings are influenced by many things in their lives, which modify their ways of thinking. Although environment, society and circle of friends influence a person to think in a certain way, the role of parents makes the ultimate significance in designing the thinking modes of a person in childhood. Till the child turns six years of age, every idea even playfully tossed by mother and father is taken in the most serious context by the child. This was symbolically stated in our scriptures, which pronounce parents as the first universe to the child.

Whatever the child perceives till the sixth year becomes the formula or modus operandi of the subconscious. For example, when a mother and father make the baby in the womb believe that the baby is created to become a mighty winner in life, then those talks enable the baby to manifest and attract words, scenes and experiences harmonious to that first thought. In due course, the child gets to know the stories of successful people, hears words of empowerment and experiences conditions and circumstances that affirm that the child is born to become a mighty winner.

Humans are naturally intelligent as per the instinct designed by Mother Nature. Just simple polishing by pregnant mothers, their husbands and families is needed to bring about the natural genius from within the baby. It starts with the practice of talking to the baby in the womb. So my request to all pregnant mothers is that if you want to impart the best life to your baby, please be careful about what you think, speak and feel when you carry a baby in your womb. Equally important is what you should not see, talk and feel, so as to avoid exposure to negative influence on the baby.

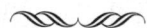

Now let us see the story of Reshma, which will portray the power of a mother's intention for her baby.

'Reshma! Reshma! What are you doing in the kitchen now?'

'Boiling milk. What do you want?'

'Shhhh . . . Come without any noise and see what our little Mukund is doing.'

'I am busy right now, Rohit.'

'You can be busy later. Here . . . I've switched off the stove. Come fast!'

'Rohit—'

'Shhh . . .'

Rohit drags Reshma along and makes her peep from behind the curtain into the room where little boy Mukund is sitting and doing something. As Reshma peeps in, she sees Mukund writing with his left hand as fluently as he would with his right hand.

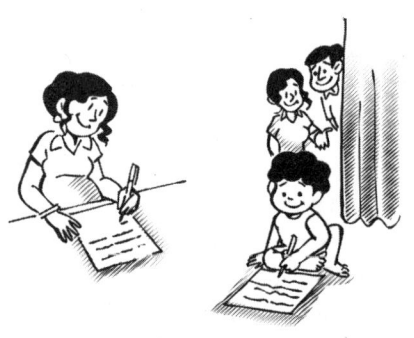

Mukund imbibing left-handed writing without being taught

Surprised, Reshma quietly enters the room with her husband in tow and slowly approaches Mukund and sits beside him. Mukund looks up at his mother and father, smiles and continues to write with his left hand. He then casually shifts the pencil from his left hand to his right hand and continues writing.

Before Rohit tries to ask Mukund something, Reshma tells him in sign language not to ask anything and lovingly hugs Mukund and leaves the room without disturbing him. Once the couple reaches the other room, Rohit speaks up in a low tone.

'Reshma, our son is writing with both hands with equal dexterity! How is it possible? Did you teach him? Should we consult the doctor?'

'Relax, Rohit, there's nothing wrong with this. In fact, a person with this ability is called ambidextrous. This ability is believed to result in higher IQ in that person.'

'But how can our son be ambidextrous when both of us are right-handed?'

'Lefties can be born to a couple who are righties. There is no abnormality in that. But I think our son being ambidextrous has something to do with what I did when Mukund was in my womb.'

'What! What did you do when you were carrying him?'

'I came to know that ambidextrous kids are high in IQ. So, I started practising writing with my left hand and in due course, I felt comfortable with it. I had a strong desire that our baby be ambidextrous with high IQ. In fact, I practised writing with my left hand, so that I can teach him left-handed writing when he grows up. I am surprised that without my teaching it, he is writing. So, the intention during pregnancy itself seems very powerful. That's the reason why today Mukund happens to have very high IQ and he learns things very fast and is praised by his teachers for his intelligence and good behaviour.'

'It is all so good, Reshma! I travel a lot and am always busy at work. Now I feel that I am missing out a lot with Mukund.'

'Actually, I have video-recorded some of the great moments I thought that you and any other important person in our life should not miss. I have started compiling a mini video of our little Mukund to gift it to the person who gave me the amazing tool of Talking to the Baby in the Womb and made my delivery easy and normal, Dr Andal!'

'Yes, Reshma. Hats off to Woman Power!'

That's the amazing power of a mother's love and intention, producing an incredible effect on the baby. It's the way of nurturing moms!

Dr Thomas Verny observes, 'If nurtured in love and kindness, your child will easily acquire these other skills when the time comes.'*

Here is yet another beautiful incident to be read and enjoyed.

'Harsha, are you sure that your teacher wants to see me?'

'Yes, Mom, I am sure she wants to see you.'

'But what did you do that she wants to meet me?'

'I didn't do anything, Mom!'

'I personally sit with you when you do your homework. What could this be all about?'

Harsha's Mom, Divya, reaches the school and meets his teacher 'Good Morning, ma'am!'

---

* Verny, *Pre-Parenting*, p. 57.

'Good morning, Mrs Divya, very nice to meet you! Please come, let's go near that tree and talk. Harsha dear, please go to class.'

'Okay, ma'am. Bye, Mom!'

'Bye, Harsha. Finish your snacks.'

'Okay, Mom.'

'Ma'am, Harsha told me that you wanted to meet me. I'm sorry for whatever mistake he may have made.'

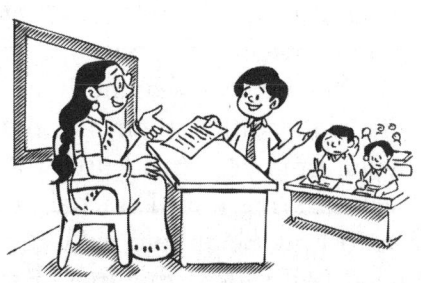

Miss, I care more about the knowledge than the marks

'Wait Divya, what made you think that Harsha must have made some mistake?'

'Thank God! I was so scared! He didn't make any mistake?'

'Trust me, Divya, Harsha is one of the best-behaved kids in the class. This is about something that is totally different. Yesterday, I gave a spell test in class as dictation. Harsha finished it very fast and handed the paper over to me. I told him to revise it once so that he could correct any mistakes. Without any hesitation, he replied in a confident tone that he was bothered more about knowledge than the marks.'

'He said that?'

'Yes. He was neither scared when he said that, nor was his tone offensive. I was somewhat taken aback because when we playfully ask the kids whether we can cut their marks for something, they usually start crying. But Harsha's reaction was the first of its kind in my experience! That's why I wanted to meet you in person and ask whether this has something to do with what you or his dad or any elder in the family who might have inspired this.'

'Ma'am, this has nothing to do with anyone in the family other than me. But you won't believe it when I tell you this. I used to talk to Harsha when I was carrying him. I started talking a lot to the baby as to how he should grow up to be a good human being with great qualities. I started telling him and reading him stories with good morals. There was this particular story of a student I used to tell him often because whenever I told him the story, Harsha used to respond from within. He used to express his liking for the story through his movements. The moral of that story was that knowledge is more important than scores.

After delivering Harsha, I got so busy bringing him up and attending to the needs of others in the family that I completely forgot about that story. I have never once narrated the story, nor have I mentioned it! But today, seven years after his birth, to hear you say that he repeated the exact words to you, I am completely surprised! I don't know what to say or how to react to this because I am very happy that my son has grasped everything I said during pregnancy and today it has influenced him in a good way!'

'Wow! Divya, you have given the best gift to your son when you were carrying him.'

'Thank you, ma'am, and I give you my word that I will see to it that Harsha revises answer sheets from now on!'

'I believe when you say this Divya, because you have already created magic with your son! Revision training will be a lot easier in comparison!'

Divya leaves with pride only a mother can feel.

We will now see the words of Dr Bruce Lipton in *The Biology of Belief,* 'The latest genetic research [suggests that] parents should cultivate that twinkle in the months before they conceive a child. That growth-promoting awareness and intention can produce a smarter, healthier and happier baby and that parents act as genetic engineers for their children in the months before conception.'*

According to Christine Homan, 'The genes are the bricks and mortar to build a brain. The environment is the architect.'

Why Are Jews So Smart?

There are lots of geniuses among the Jews. Nearly one-fourth of Nobel Prize scientists are Jews! Albert Einstein, Sigmund Freud and Karl Marx were all Jews!

---

* Lipton. *Biology of Belief,* p. 142.

It is observed that Israelis begin their preparation from pregnancy. Israeli mothers make conscious efforts to play the piano and solve mathematical problems together with their husbands. They practise this diligently as they strongly believe that this will help them give birth to genius kids. Pregnant women regularly eat almonds, dates and fish. Israeli culture makes it obligatory for pregnant women to consume cod liver oil. In Israel, people are against smoking. Scientists have demonstrated that nicotine has the potential to destroy brain cells and affect the genes, resulting in generations of moronic or defective brain. Right from childhood, children are given compulsory training in playing the piano or the violin. They believe that this practice increases the IQ of the child and makes him a genius. According to Jewish scientists, the vibration of the music stimulates the brain.

Brain Growth

The brain size of a baby at birth is almost 30 per cent of an adult's brain size, but its body weight is only 5 per cent of an adult's. Up to 80 per cent of the brain's growth occurs during the first two years. Promotion of breastfeeding enhances brain growth. Breastfed babies have at least eight points higher intelligence quotient in later life as compared to formula-fed babies. The remaining 20 per cent of brain growth occurs during pre-school years wherein special attention needs to be paid to complementary feeds and optimal intake of micronutrients consisting of vitamins and trace minerals. By twenty-eight weeks of pregnancy (seventh month) all the vital senses, the vision, hearing, taste, touch and smell are functional. Of them, touch and hearing are very well developed. Memory tracts are laid down from twenty-eight weeks. Learning and memory develop in the third trimester. When there is happiness, the memory is retained for a long time. This shows a baby can learn in the womb and remember it well in later life. This is a typical example of unconscious memory, called implicit memory.

At birth, connections per neuron (nerve cell) are 2500, but by age two or three, it's about 15,000 per neuron, twice as many as adults. Forming and reinforcing these connections (wiring) are the key tasks of early brain development. Most of this wiring is completed in the first two to three years. Wiring helps build either a strong and supportive, or a fragile and unreliable foundation.

How are connections (wiring) formed and deleted? Loving interactions with caring adults strongly stimulate a child's brain, causing synapses (connections) to grow and existing connections to get stronger. Touching, holding, comforting, rocking, singing, and talking to them provide the best kind of stimulation for their growing brains and for their emotional security. Stress reduces the connections. High stress during pregnancy can result in lower IQ scores. These connections, when they are not used, are lost. Intelligence can be developed by taking specific nutrients and stimulation measures. Nutrients for the brain: omega-3 fatty acid, Docosahexaenoic acid (DHA), vitamin B complex, folic acid, vitamin C, vitamin E, iodine, iron, zinc, selenium and essential amino acids including taurine and Choline.

Healthy Eating

In order to get a healthy and intelligent baby, expectant mothers should take healthy foods that provide a lot of nutrients. Deficiency of iron, iodine and other minerals may cause learning disabilities, language development problems, and delayed development of motor skills, lower IQ and even behavioural problems in the babies. Iodine is essential for making thyroid hormones, which are essential for the development of the brain. Iron is essential for making red blood cells, which carry oxygen to different parts of the mother's body and to the baby. Choline is vital for brain development, especially the parts associated with recall and memory.

Folic acid

Pregnant women should get at least 400 micrograms of folic acid daily from their food or other supplements. It is ideal to take folic acid at least one month prior to conception to lower the risks of brain and spinal cord defects. Citrus fruits, broccoli, liver, green leafy vegetables, beans, etc. are good sources of folic acid.

DHA

DHA is an omega-3 fatty acid that plays a crucial role in significantly improving the intelligence of the baby. Omega-3 fatty acids are available from fatty fish such as tuna, salmon, herring and fish oil. Flax seeds and walnuts are good vegetarian sources.

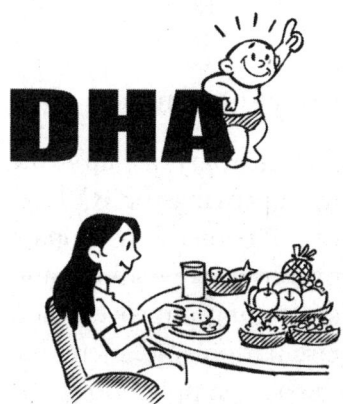

For intelligence

DHA supplements are available too. Those healthy fats provide faster development, and healthier nerve connections.

Importance of Breast-Feeding

Breastfeeding is best for brain growth and neuromotor development of the babies. Human milk contains thirty times more DHA (omega-3 fatty acid) than cow's milk. Human milk is rich in choline, taurine and zinc, which are essential for brain growth.

Expectant mothers should gain healthy weight during this period as low weight gain results in delivering of low-weight babies and experts say that the IQ of a baby and its birth weight are positively correlated up to eight pounds of birth weight. Hence healthy eating and weight gain are essential to improve the IQ of the baby in the womb.

Exercise to Improve IQ

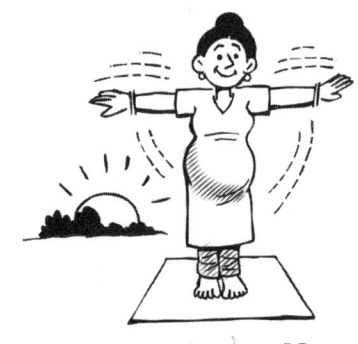

Exercise to increase IQ

Exercise plays a major role in improving the IQ level of a foetus. Low-impact exercises like walking and swimming improve blood circulation and increased nutrient supply boosts the brain development. After five months of pregnancy, mothers can rock gently and slowly in a rocking chair several times a day. It is likely to enhance neuromotor development and coordination ability of the baby.

Reduce Stress

The amount of stress the expecting mother may have during her pregnancy affects the development of the baby because chronic stress produces a hormone called cortisol, which affects the baby. Some research indicates that high stress during pregnancy can result in lower IQ scores. Pregnant women can try journal writing, taking plenty of naps, reading to the baby, soaking their feet for relaxation, meditation and yoga.

Stimulation

Babies have a biological need to learn. Any stimulation through his special senses of hearing, sight, taste, smell and touch provided during foetal life and preschool years has a profound effect on the growth and maturation of brain. It has been shown that a stimulation programme can promote faster growth, improve coordination of muscular movements, increase span of concentration and raise the baby's IQ by as much as fifteen points. Hearing and touch are well developed for the baby in the womb.

Talking to the Baby in the Womb

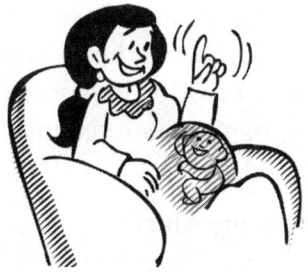

Talking to the Baby in the Womb to be smart

Babies can recognize sounds even when they are in the womb. Hence, talk to them and let them realize how much you love baby. Loving manner has positive effects on their memory and emotions, building the foundations of language. The mother should give positive suggestions to her baby whenever she is in a relaxed mood and before going to sleep. The foetus is alert during the evening. Also, make the baby listen to the voice of the father, siblings and other family members and this will create a positive effect on the emotion and language development of the baby.

Story Time with Baby

Reading stories aloud to the baby during pregnancy has advantages; it is a useful bonding experience. It also encourages the cognitive development of the baby. Pregnant women need to choose a relaxing and quiet place and suitable time and make it a daily routine. They can

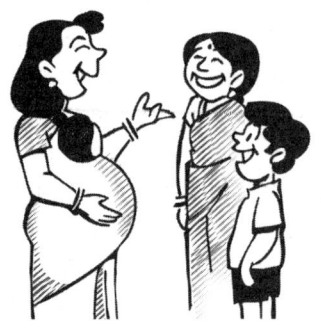

Family members talking to baby

select stories from scriptures, verses, autobiographies of great people, moral stories, which they can tell again as bedtime stories when the baby grows up. Choosing books that utilize repetition, rhyming and rhythm can help stimulate cognitive development, pattern recognition and language skills in the children.

Playing Music

The latest data shows that music and language are so intertwined that an awareness of music is critical to a baby's language development. As children grow, music fosters communication skills. Our sense of song helps them learn to talk, read and even make friends. A study of musicians' brains shows over five times as many interconnections in the brain as non-musicians. Student musicians have an average of eleven points higher in IQ than non-musicians.

Touch to Boost IQ

Pregnant women can experience the movements of the baby from the fifth month of pregnancy and by the seventh or eighth month, the movements become very clear and the mother can feel the kicks and jerks of the baby. If we keenly observe, we will notice certain parts of the baby such as feet, palm or head clearly over the abdomen. This is the best time we can connect with the baby in the womb as the baby can also feel the touch. This stimulates the baby's brain to search for more sensations and thus improves sensory skills.

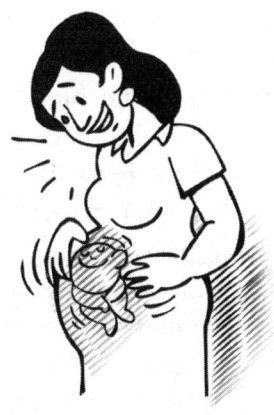

Touch to boost IQ

Research also suggests that this type of stimulation is relaxing and reassuring for the baby. The baby will often respond to this stimulation by kicking or pushing back.

Have Your Baby When You Are Young

The age of father and mother also plays a significant role in determining the intelligence of their baby.

Avoid Alcohol and Smoking

Expecting mothers who have the smoking habit are more likely to have a less intelligent baby as the smoke constricts the blood vessels and reduces the flow of blood to the foetus, thereby reducing the availability of the nutrients, which affects the brain cells that are essential for the cognitive development of the baby. Even passive smoking is considered dangerous for the baby. Alcohol consumption is more dangerous as alcohol intoxicates the baby and causes poor IQ, cognitive skills, poor memory, poor reasoning, attention deficits, etc. If intoxication is much higher, then it may even lead to permanent damage to the brain and central nervous system.

The process of talking to the baby in the womb as a way of stimulating the brain must be continued even after birth to reap the benefits. IQ and EQ can be developed from childhood.

EQ (Emotional Quotient)

EQ includes creativity, perseverance and, perhaps most important, flexibility and self-control. This can be consciously developed by attentive and committed parents. EQ helps in improving IQ. According to Prof. Anne Fernald, children developed language best when their parents talked about things children found interesting. She said plunking a child in front of the television or giving an iPad to play with was no substitute for a conversation that centred on the child and its interests, and might even have damaging effects on the children's language development. She said, 'You are obligated to feed them, wash them, and clothe them. Talk to them while you are doing it. We are not saying quit your job and homeschool them.'

Studies on babies and toddlers found that striking differences emerged in their vocabularies and language processing skills as early as eighteen months old.

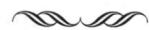

Confucius: A Chinese Philosopher

The mother of Confucius was Yen Ching-tsai. K'ung Ho was an older man, perhaps seventy years old. His first wife had died, leaving him the father of nine daughters. But K'ung Ho also hoped to have a son and married Yen Ching-tsai. Yen Ching tsai travelled to Ni-ch'iu Mountain and prayed for a son. That night, she dreamed that a spirit had come to her and said, 'You shall have a son, who will be a great sage and prophet, and you must bring him forth

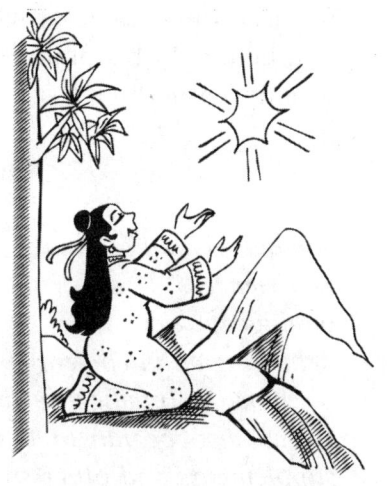

Confucius's mother, Ching-tsai

in the hollow mulberry tree.' Not long after this, she became pregnant. During the pregnancy, she had a vision of a carved prophecy: 'The son of the essence of water shall soon succeed to the withering Chou, and be a throne-less king'; which meant that her baby would grow up to become a wise and valued leader. At the time of birth, Ching-tsai heard music, and a voice saying to her: 'Heaven is moved at the birth of your son, and sends down harmonious sounds.' A spring of water bubbled up within the dry cave so that Ching-tsai could bathe her new baby and to confirm the prophecy that the new baby was the 'son of the essence of water.' Confucius is said to have worked as a governor of a town in the Lu Kingdom in 501 BC. Some accounts say that when he was sixty-eight years old, he taught his philosophy to about sixty-eight or seventy-seven disciples.

Sahana: Thanks, Aunty, for sharing such amazing experiences. I am confident about delivering an intelligent kid. What is your success mantra for delivering an intelligent child.

Doctor: Intelligence can be in nature (hereditary). It can also be nurtured with strong intention, diet, supplements and other stimulatory activities; it is not entirely dependent on the educational status of the parents, but on the emotional commitment. Later, it can be honed with persuasion. When coupled with right conduct, it yields fruitful results.

Sahana: Perfect, Aunty, I got the message. I'll start practising it right away.

Arjun: I understood that keeping mother and baby happy will surely make the baby intelligent. This is in sync with happy schooling in Finland. Finnish students are known to be toppers in PISA (Program for International Student Assessment). I feel intelligence and morality are like two eyes. I'll also discuss this with Sahana and my mother so that they will be amicable partners in grooming the baby.

Doctor: Arjun, you have made the whole concept crystal-clear! Come let's have dinner.

After dinner

Arjun: Aunty, may I leave now? Thanks a lot for the valuable information and sumptuous dinner. I'll learn from Sahana about other aspects of Talking to the Baby in the Womb.

Doctor: Okay, Arjun, Sahana. Next, we'll talk about moulding the behaviour of the baby, which is my favourite topic. Bye, for now!

Sahana: Okay, Aunty. Bye! Good night.

Teacher asked me to write essay on dog.

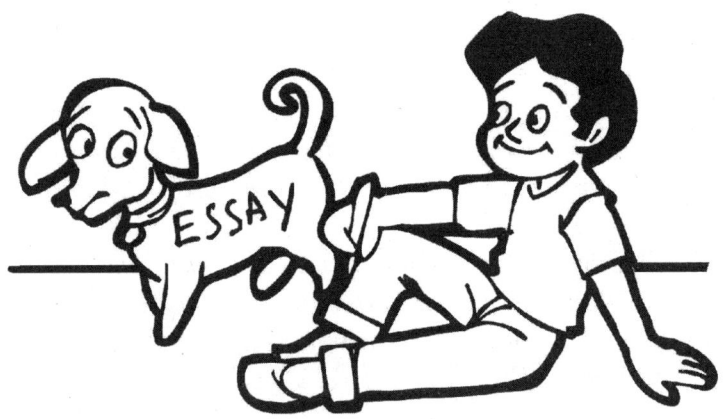

5

Behaviour Modification

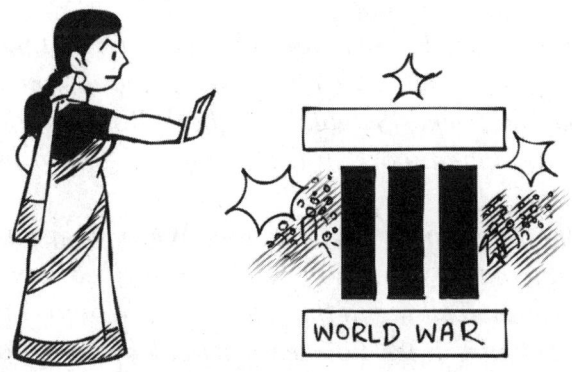

Men cannot stop the Third World War. It is not in their cells. But women can. The solutions on this Earth are in the hands of the woman, in the psyche of the woman.

—**Yogi Bhajan**

When motherhood becomes the fruit of a deep yearning, not the result of ignorance or accident, its children will become the foundation of a new race.

—Margaret Sanger

Sahana: Aunty! Here's yet another student for Talking to the Baby. My dad, Mr Shankar, the famous educationist, promoting the 'happy-schooling concept'. Mom and Dad are excited about Talking to the Baby. He wants to listen to you talk about his pet subject—value-based education.

Doctor: Hello! Shankar. Though I'm meeting you for the first time, I've heard a lot about you from Vijaya, my friend [Sahana's mother]. Both of you are doing dedicated work in education and I'm proud of you both.

Shankar: Same here, madam. We have a passion for value-based education. We were thrilled when we heard about Talking to the Baby in the Womb concept from Sahana. I see how easy it will be to groom a designer baby produced through Talking to the Baby in the Womb, because what we do in our work, is just trying to redo or re-educate; it takes a lot of energy and patience to re-educate both parents and students. In one masterstroke, you are programming great personalities, easily and effectively. You are sowing seeds, and we are watering.'

Doctor: Wow, great Shankar! You are able to see the connect. There can't be a better example. I'm glad about it.

Sahana: Now, Aunty, will you tell us about moulding the behaviour of the baby in the womb?

Doctor: Yes, Sahana! Motherhood is a status for society, but it's a moral responsibility executed with love for parents, particularly a mother. We can observe a strong connection between how you respond to certain situations during your pregnancy and how the child is going to respond to similar situations after birth. Let me share some of the experiences. We will see the friendship of Mallika with little Rohan.

Mallika: 'Rohan, I was just thinking of you and here you are, my dear boy! Why are you late to play with me today?'

'Mom gave me raddu to eat, that's why.' 'What are you doing with the slippers, Rohan?'

'I am keeping them in order.'

'Oh, that's a very good habit. I know that the slippers were strewn all over the place. You have arranged them neatly! Super! Okay, coming back to the topic, you said that you ate raddu? What is that?'

'Don't you know raddu? Yellow and round, see! I brought some for you also.'

'Oh, you mean laddu?'

'Yes, laddu.'

'Ha, ha! I love the way you pronounce laddu as raddu. Thanks for getting it for me. Very, very thoughtful of you, Rohan.'

Rohan's mother, Geeta, comes in. 'Hello, Mallika! I have brought some Laddus for you to relish.'

'Hi, Geetha akka. Please come. Thank you very much. But I must tell you that these days I enjoy raddus more than laddus.'

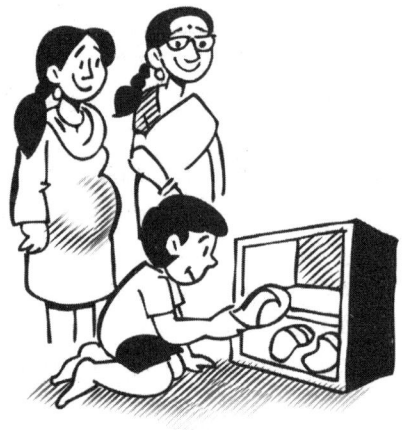

Rohan carefully arranges the slippers

'Haha! Rohan, what is the name of the cow that came to our house this morning?'

'Rakshmi.'

Mallika repeats, 'Rakshmi?'

'He is just three years old. He pronounces L as R. Laddus become raddus and Lakshmi is rakshmi for him. We are training him in the correct pronunciation of L.'

'Oh, I am just enjoying the innocence of Rohan's pronunciations. Let it be raddu and rakshmi for us. The baby talk is divine. It will vanish in a year or so. Please don't correct him now, akka.'

This is how Mallika loves to remember her little friend Rohan. Mallika, while talking to her baby, tells it to be as smart, loving and sharing as her little friend

Rohan. Time runs by. It has been over three years since those days. Now Mallika is the mother of a smart and loving two-year-old boy Ajay, and she lives in Bengaluru.

'Hello, Mrs Mallika, how are you?'

'Thank you, Mrs Sarojini, I am doing very well. How is Ajay performing? I hope he behaves well with his classmates.'

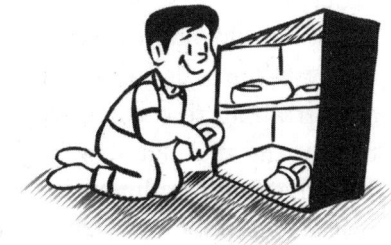

Ajay does it exactly like Rohan

'Mrs Mallika, I must tell you that your son Ajay is the best-behaved kid in the class. He is very smart and his most striking quality is that he shares his stationery and snacks with everyone, even with me. He has a big heart and generous spirit. I wanted to ask you as to what you did to train Ajay to be this bright? His childish talks are very endearing as well. Today being our annual day, we distributed sweets to the children. It's laddus. When I gave it to Ajay, he said, 'Thank you, ma'am, I just love raddus!'

'What? He said that?'

'Yes, he calls his friend Lakshmi as rakshmi. Haha! His childish talks are so sweet to hear . . .'

The surprised Mallika recollects the days she enjoyed with her little friend Rohan, their tenant's son, during her pregnancy when she was at her mother's place. She remembers how she wanted her baby to be just like Rohan, smart, loving and giving.

Mallika is at home with her son. She finishes her work in the kitchen and comes to see what Ajay is doing and she finds Ajay arranging his shoes neatly in order, which is so like his favourite Rohan!

So striking are the results of the Talking to the Baby in the Womb technique. The baby in the womb takes cues from all that is enjoyed by the mother and adapts to suit the mannerisms of the people she admires. So sensitive and intelligent is the baby in the womb! They just have to be wholeheartedly requested to be like someone and they never disappoint after they come into this world. When it is told with love and affection, in a state of joy and happiness, it is recorded deeply in the subconscious mind of the baby, to be played exactly as it is at the appropriate time after birth.

We observe, though not with the sophistication of an adult, the foetus feels every feeling and emotion. Dr Verny says, Dr Verny argued in *The Secret Life of the Unborn Child* that what the unborn child feels in the womb helps shape his later emotional and behavioural dispositions—whether he grows up happy or anxious, secure or shy, can depend in part on the

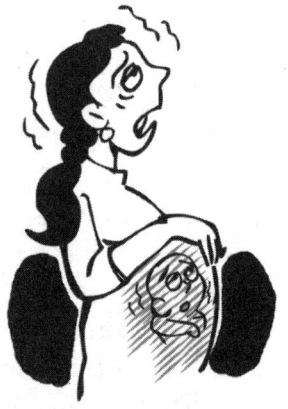

Mother's feeling is also felt by the unborn baby

emotional messages he received prenatally., in part on the messages he gets about himself in the womb'.[*]

So, it is the responsibility of the mother, father and their circles to ensure that the baby in the womb receives all the good messages.

There is well-established research indicating that maternal emotional well-being during pregnancy—covering stress, anxiety and mood disturbances—can significantly influence birth outcomes. Maternal mental health issues in the third trimester are linked to pre-term birth and low birth weight, indicating that poor mental health is a clear risk factor.[†]

In a large cohort study, mothers who experienced psychological distress—such as anxiety and depression—had babies with lower birth weight and impaired fetal growth.[‡] Another personal experience of mine would be with Sneha.

Sneha delivered a baby that kept crying incessantly and would become jittery even at the slightest noise. All the tests were normal. Many doctors saw the baby. Finally, one senior paediatrician suggested that they should not allow anyone into the room where the baby was. Everyone must be cautious enough not to make any noise. Regular bath was avoided and gentle sponge

---

[*] Verny with Kelly. *The Secret Life*.
[†] Huang, Qingyu, Tingting Sun, et al. 'Association of Maternal Mental Health with Neonatal Outcomes: A Prospective Cohort Study in China', *Frontiers in Public Health*, Vol. 10 (2022).
[‡] Goedhart, Gerda, Vrijkotte, Vincent W., et al. 'Maternal Psychological Distress during Pregnancy and Fetal Growth Restriction: The ABCD Study', *American Journal of Clinical Nutrition*, Vol. 90, no. 3 (2009), pp. 626–32.

bath with a towel was given. Slowly, the baby's cry subsided after a few weeks. When Sneha was made to open up her mind and speak, she came out with the root cause of this problem.

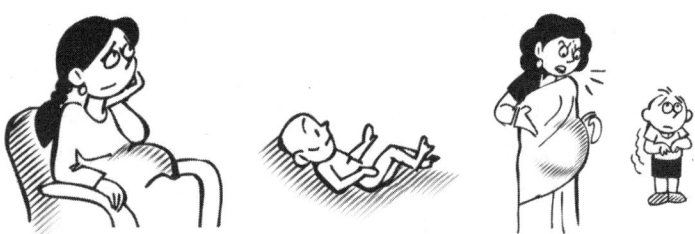

When mother is anxious and worried, baby will be irritable, restless and jittery with frequent crying.

During her pregnancy, she was very anxious and always feared harm to the baby. She kept her hands on her abdomen to protect the baby, even while walking. The baby took cue from her feelings and became insecure, timid and jittery even at the slightest noise and cried.

Suggestions to Mothers Who Suffer Negative Thinking

If you have continuous negative thinking or tendencies, please try to understand that there is one or more serious

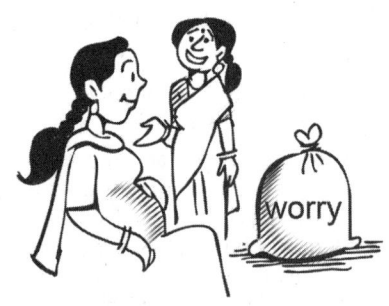

Talking to a friend helps unburden worry.

core beliefs that are related to that thought pattern. This pattern surfaces as a warning in the form of tendencies and emotions. When these tendencies are not taken care of or not addressed properly, they start showing up as disease and discomfort. It is important to note that physical symptoms can have a mental root cause. But also remember that there is no need to panic. All you need to do is talk to yourself and your baby. Have someone as your support system or a tracker system.

The first step is for you to open up to that person, confide and pour out all that presses your mind and feelings. And once the cause is known, the solution will be the next logical order. With the help of the person who is your support system, you can find the right solution and, in the meantime, erase the cause and replace it with positivity and optimistic feelings and emotions. Then allow your trackers to take care. This means, allow the person who is your biggest support system to make sure that you are in the right mode and pattern of thinking all that is good for your health first and also that of your baby. Once the pressing, pressurizing issue is erased, you will turn out to be the member of the 'ideal mom' category with ease and peace.

If you practise the Talking to the Baby in the Womb technique well, it helps you to come out of negative feelings quite easily. You can also ask for help from the baby to understand and cooperate with you; and the baby is sure to oblige when the bond is based on love, and not on doubt. Life loves you and so does your baby. So, do what is right, safe and healthy for the baby not only physically but also mentally.

According to Goodlatte, 'there are two primary focuses that you can practice. One is to create a more calm and happy you, the other is to create a more happy and healthy child. This can be done in just a few minutes each day. In a place that is free of interruptions, simply close your eyes and practise seeing, feeling and even hearing a healthy baby. Conjure as many senses as you can, as feeling may be more important than seeing. Use the richness of your imagination, and start daydream. If other thoughts enter your mind, patiently return to your happy self and healthy baby. Like actors who develop emotions on cue, practicing positive thoughts and feelings will branch neurons and wire parts of your brain to respond accordingly. The more you practice, the faster and better you will you learn to retrieve those emotions.'[*]

This is yet another case that shows how mother's desire is exactly and effortlessly carried out by the child after birth.

'I want to go home . . .'

Some of the young kids at the day care centre are crying as they miss their mothers. Many kids look at the crying kids and they start crying as well.

'Children, please don't cry, in about an hour, your parents will be here to pick you up. Come, let us

---

[*] Goodlatte, James. 'A Mother's Emotions Affects Her Unborn Child' (*Epoch Times,* 14 January 2014), https://www.theepochtimes.com/article/a-mothers-emotions-affect-her-unborn-child-435739, accessed on 11 July 2025.

all listen to a story or would you like to listen to a song?'

'Snacks for all!'

'Here comes the snacks trolley! Come on, all of you!'

'I don't want snacks. I want to go to my mommy.'

'I don't want any story or song, I want to go to my granny, take me home now!'

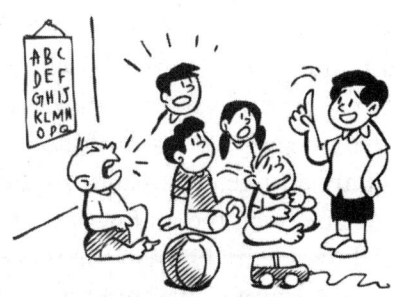

Nishchint talks to the other kids in a clear voice

'Oh God! What shall we do now, Kumar?'

'Ma'am, this is the daily fear that we go through; around this time, the kids start missing their mothers and grandmothers and they all start crying.'

'Nishchint is the only boy who never cries. He is always calm.'

'See there, Nishchint is going and standing up in front of the kids as if to say something, let's hear what he is up to.'

Nishchint talks in a clear voice to the other kids.

'Hey, why are you all crying? I want to go home too! But till the bell rings and our parents or grandparents are here, Bhanu ma'am and Kumar bhaiya will not allow us to go home. They are not going to send us home without our elders. Then, what is the point in you people crying?'

The kids somehow stop crying and become quiet. They all start eating snacks and start playing together. When his mother Amrutha comes to pick him up, Bhanu and Kumar ask her the secret behind Nishchint's calmness. Amrutha reveals the secret as follows. 'When I was pregnant with Nishchint, I observed my sister's son cry for everything and never give anything to anyone. I used to tell Nischinth not to be a 'crybaby'. He should never cry unnecessarily and should always remain calm and composed. I also wanted him to be a smart and generous kid, friendly with all. So, he took the cue from me and now I am enjoying the benefits of talking to my baby in the womb. He has turned out to be everything I wanted him to be! Talking to the Baby in the Womb does all the miracles!'

The womb is the first world of the baby. The environment created for the experiences of the baby inside the womb creates the baby's personality and character predispositions. If the womb environment is welcoming, kind, loving and warm, the baby is likely to expect the outside world to be similar. This creates a trust, openness, character of extroversion and self-confidence in the baby's attitude towards the self and the world.

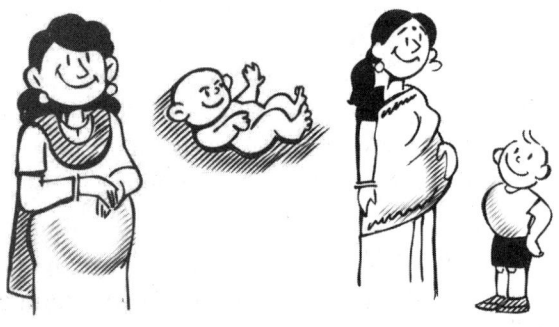

When mom is happy, baby will be healthy and happy after birth

We'll see it being reflected in the attitude of little Dharani.

For Sowmya, it was a precious pregnancy. She had conceived five years after marriage. She would always pray that the baby would be a gift to her and her adorable family. She was talking to her baby in the womb and developed a rapport with it. She was sharing her dreams about the baby, a valuable gift she was passing on to the family. As her daughter Dharani grew up, she found her to be doting on her; helping her in kitchen, doing small errands unasked. Her grandfather would feel happy when the little one spontaneously fetched him a glass of water as soon as he returned home. He used to tell his son, 'I am least bothered about you all. It's enough if my little Dharani is with me.'

Sowmya's husband feels proud of his daughter because whenever the family would go out she would insist he give alms to beggars. He would say, 'I don't think there can be a better girl than my daughter.' Sowmya felt her dream was fulfilled. It was the mother's desire that influenced the personality, resulting in unfolding of performance and skills in different activities.

In his book, *The Secret Life of the Unborn Child,* Dr Verny recorded yet another incident about the behaviour of young children as follows:

'It can be found in the rural areas of Africa where women carry their newborns, sack-like, on their back or slung on to their sides. Held either way, a baby can easily soil his mother's clothes with his bowel and bladder eliminations. But this almost never happens to an African mother. Somehow she is able to sense his urges in enough time to swing him off her back and hold him away from her before he eliminates. This form of intuitive knowledge is hardly considered unusual. In fact, an African woman soiled by her child after his seventh day of life is loudly and widely branded a poor mother.'

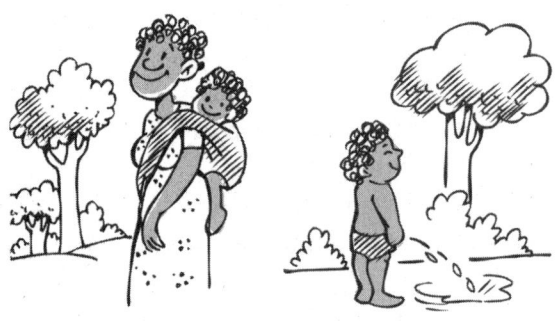

In Africa's tribal village, babies don't soil mother's clothes

One of our mothers, Pavithra and her husband Shiva were talking to the baby during pregnancy and after birth. They asked the baby not to urinate in the bed. The baby alerts them with a cooing sound and the mother immediately attends to her. The parents are very proud about their understanding daughter.

The moulding of behaviour can be seen at the country level. Emile Coue explains this in Spartan and Athens mothers.

Emile Coue, a French psychologist and psychotherapist, popularized a method called conscious autosuggestion. Let's see what he has to say about mental preparation of a mother during pregnancy.

> It may seem paradoxical but, nevertheless, the education of a child ought to begin before its birth. In sober truth, if a woman, a few weeks after conception, makes a mental picture of the child she is going to bring forth into the world, of the physical and moral qualities with which she desires to see it endowed and if she will continue during the time of gestation to impress on herself the same mental image, the child will have the qualities desired. Spartan women only brought forth robust children, who grew to be redoubtable warriors, because their strongest desire was to give such heroes to their country; whilst, at Athens, mothers had intellectual children whose mental qualities were a hundred-fold greater than their physical attributes.*

Coue's autosuggestion seems to have been proved correct in our country during the freedom struggle.

Freedom Fighters during the Indian Independence Struggle

Try to recall the days of the Indian independence struggle. Women at that time must have realized that the sole purpose of life was to serve the country. They must

---

* 'Day By Day in Every Way I Am Getting Better and Better: Emile Coué and the Birth of American Positive Thinking (Unpublished 1972)', The Life and Media of Gordon F. Sander, https://www.gordonsander.com/day-by-day, accessed on 22 August 2025.

have been imbued with the spirit of freedom by having patriotic men as fathers, brothers and husbands. They must have thought that the only way they could serve the nation was by giving birth to patriotic children. Among those who belonged to this category were the mothers of Mahatma Gandhi (Putlibai), Jawaharlal Nehru (Swaruprani), and Sardar Vallabhabai Patel (Laad Bai). They all had high regards for their mothers. They were all selfless, upright, honest, and committed leaders and led a life of sacrifice. In that period, leaders of such qualities emerged in different parts of the country.

When the mother's desire was so strong, there was every possibility that she would give birth to a son or daughter with desired qualities. Swamy Vivekananda, the spiritual giant who also had a patriotic fervour, recalled, that the seed of spirituality in him was sown by his mother by way of prayers and fasting for two to three years before his birth.

As time passed, women thought they themselves could participate in the freedom struggle. This determination resulted in the birth of prominent leaders such as Sarojini Devi, Kamaladevi Chattopadhyay, Kalpana Dutt and Madame Bhikaji Cama.

This only goes to prove that pregnancy is not just a nine-month wait for the big event of birth but a crucial period unto itself—the staging ground for well-being, disease and unfolding of personality in later life.

Motherhood is an inherent gift. The sense of motherhood can be identified in some, right from childhood, like the ones who are just three or four years old and can still take very good care of babies younger than themselves. Some women instinctively love any child they come across. This quality is that of a nurturer. When the right messages of love and care are sent to the babies in the womb, the babies are born with amazing personalities that bring success and fame to the world as well as to their mothers. These are the wonderful gifts of nurturing moms! Hats off to them!

Let us see what Dr Thomas Verny says in this regard.

'The future of the world may well depend on how successful we are at promulgating this simple but vital message: As you do unto your own children, they will do unto the world. Children learn from what parents say and do and this is referred to as modelling. Children conceived in love, nurtured in love and born and raised with love, grow up in a state of grace and return to society many times more than what they received. To preclude violent behavior in children, parents must be aware of the following things.

Continual fighting between spouses will predispose a child to violent behavior, verbal abuse and emotional neglect can cause more psychiatric difficulty than physical battering. Watching violence on television will increase the chances of the child becoming violent himself.'*

---

* Verny with Kelly. *The Secret Life.*

Prahlada

Hiranyakashipu and Hiranyaksha were twins (demon kings) of great strength.

When Hiranyakashipu learned about the death of his brother, he became very sad and angry. He consoled his brother's wife and his own wife and left the palace to perform penance to invoke Lord Brahma and get extraordinarily special boons in order to make himself invincible. He entrusted the kingdom to his ministers. Devendra laid siege to the capital and had an easy victory. He took Hiranyakashipu's wife queen Kayadhu as a prisoner. Narada consoled Kayadhu and took her to his ashram.

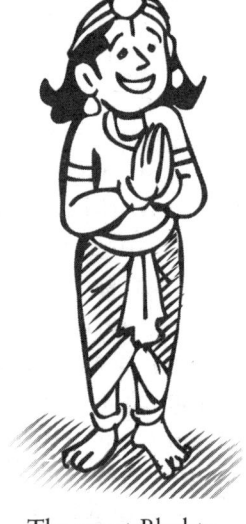

The great Bhakta Prahlada for whose sake God took Narasimha avatar

Kayadhu, the pregnant wife of Hiranyakashipu, thus began to spend a happy and contented life in sage Narada's ashram. Sage Narada would call her and talk to her privately and initiate her to noble ideas. Sometimes, while listening to the sage she would fall sleep, but sage Narada would continue his discourse and the child in her womb would listen to him with great devotion. The child would try to understand the inner meaning of his discourses. In the course of time, the child remembered even the last syllable of what he had said. After birth, the child was named Prahlada.

Prahlada was the youngest among Hiranyakashipu's four sons. He had full control over his senses, mind and body. Since childhood, he remained submerged in devotion to Lord Vishnu. Hiranyakashipu considered Lord Srihari as his archenemy. So, he tortured Prahlada by throwing him down the cliff, getting him stamped on by an elephant, burning him with fire, etc, But all these heinous acts were in vain. Nothing could harm the great devotee.

Later, the Lord burst forth from a pillar in the form of Narasimha (half man, half lion) to fulfil the word of his devotee Prahlada, and killed Hiranyakashipu. We are proud that our ancestors could produce a great devotee by infusing devotion in the womb.

Sahana: Thanks for sharing such wonderful stories, Aunty. Shankar: Let me share my conclusion, ladies.

Conscious parenting = thoughtful parenting. The mind and heart of parents must resonate to the needs of the child. Challenges of parenting make the parents feel exhausted.

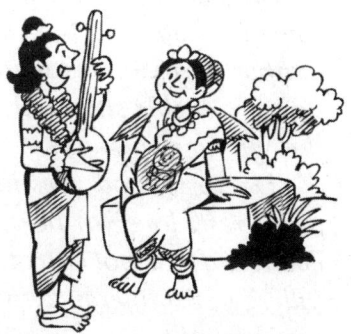

Sage Narada giving sermon during pregnancy to Kayadhu, mother of Prahalad.

Hence awareness plus mastery of a parenting tool will help. Talking to the Baby in the Womb is the master parenting tool.

The way you dress, the way you speak to other people, the way you express joy or sadness, the way you treat your friends and enemies, the way you laugh and read the newspaper, all this means a lot to the child.

Our forefathers wisely laid down certain codes of conduct in the name of culture, tradition and rituals and ensured continuation of certain behavioural traits for centuries.

Doctor: Shankar, your understanding of behaviour is awesome! I think, the continuity of Talking to the Baby in the Womb will be perfect if they admit the kid to your school

Shankar: That's exactly my feeling, as it's easier to build strong children than to repair broken men.

Sahana: Aunty, one last question, I've seen my cousin's baby keeps crying non-stop, making the mother miserable; is there anything I need to prepare to avoid such a situation or just Talking to the Baby in the Womb is enough?

Doctor: Good question, Sahana. Baby may cry for food, rest, love (to be caressed), comfort (for nappy change, if it is hot or cold),colic, pain in the abdomen (allergy or intolerance to something in breast milk, or formula milk, wind, constipation or reflux) or because it is unwell through unique cues: movement, gestures, sound and facial expressions. This crying is probably just a phase. As your baby grows, he or she will learn new ways of communicating its needs to you. And when this happens, the excessive crying will soon stop.

Sahana: Are there any specific suggestions for mothers to groom children as happy and righteous individuals?

Doctor: Mothers are mentally conditioned only for joy and celebration with baby; not for exhaustion, anxiety and responsibility. They need to be mentally and physically well prepared, so that they can be relaxed and have a beneficial influence on the child.

Sahana: Thank you so much, Aunty. As you said, the mother's mental preparation to handle the baby is an important parenting tip.

Shankar: Ma'am, you please visit our school.

Doctor: Sure, Shankar. I'll visit the school. In fact, I want to see the effect of sports and music on schoolchildren. We'll also interact with the children, and see how introduction of music during pregnancy plays an integral role in happiness, health and intelligence.

Live so that your children think of fairness, caring and integrity when they think of you.

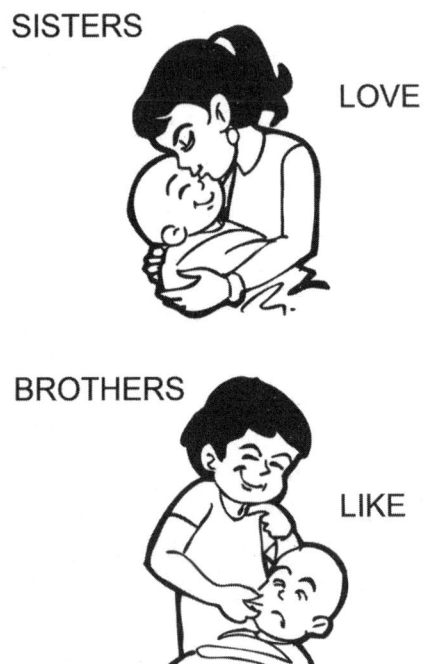

6

The Tunes of Life

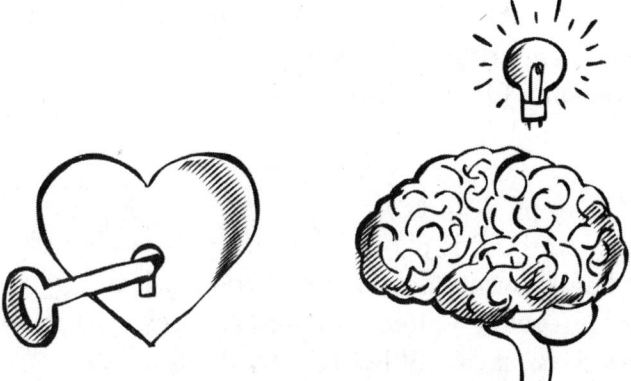

Music is the magical key that opens the heart and activates the brain; brings tenderness and warmth into the heart and light and freedom into the mind.

Shankar: Hello, Doctor, welcome to our eco cottage. Let's go round the school. Vijaya is out of station and she will catch up with you later.

We'll go to Shanthi Kuteer, our meditation hut. You will feel a calming effect listening to the music at 432 Hz, which resonates with the heartbeat of Mother Earth.

Doctor: Amazing!

After coming out of the hut, the doctor says: Yes, Shankar. It's very peaceful, calming the mind and relaxing the body. It's good you are providing such a wonderful experience to teachers and children.

Sahana: Aunty, will you tell us about the effect of music during pregnancy?

Doctor: Yes, Sahana, listen to the interesting story, the influence of womb song.

Suhana: Okay, Aunty.

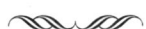

'Shiva Stotram' is played and Tripura's mother places her hands on her daughter's abdomen. It is Tripura's third pregnancy after two miscarriages. Her family takes the best care of her and her unborn baby.

'Yes, the baby is doing well in your womb, Tripura.'

'Mom, you have a way of finding out the well-being of the baby.' Tripura's sister Indhu comes and speaks with love.

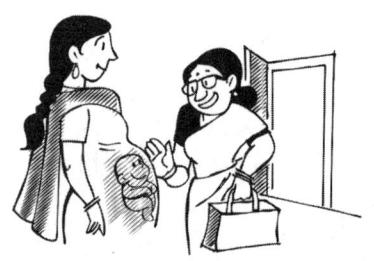

Tripura's mom talking to the baby, counting the movements.

'Hey sis, can I talk to my godchild for a bit?'

'You are most welcome, Indhu! Why would you need any permission for that?'

'Hey, my darling, inside my loving sister's womb, how are you today? How was the lunch your grandma cooked for you? Did you enjoy it?'

Tripura's sister Indhu feels the movement of the baby in her sister's tummy and smiles.)

'Oh, you just loved the taste? I am so happy you liked it. You know what? I have planted a small mango tree in our garden. After you come out, safe and healthy, we will water the tree together and when the tree gives the sweetest of Banganappalli mangoes, we shall both sit under the tree and enjoy them. Okay? Then I wanted to tell you this. My friend Ramya's dog has delivered nine pups. They are all healthy and chubby. We'll see them later. I will take you to the zoo as you grow up a bit. There you can see all forest animals and birds as well. You have to eat well, sleep well, drink enough milk and stay healthy. Only then can we do a lot of adventurous things together. Hey, here comes your grandpa. He is going to play you your favourite song; enjoy the song and rest a bit, I will catch up with you in a while, love you.'

Tripura's father walks into the room.

'Now it's my turn to play the songs for my grandchild. You ladies take rest. Hey, my darling grandchild. First, I will play you your favourite film song. Tripura, you please let me know how the baby is enjoying the song.'

'Sure, Dad! Play on!'

The song plays. Tripura and her mom feel the baby's movements. Tripura's mom giggles and speaks.

'The baby thoroughly enjoys the song! He or she is literally dancing to the tune! It is party time now in there.'

'My darling, super cool! This is how I want my grandchild to remember me, once it steps into this world. I want to be one of the closest and best friends with my grandchild! This is the least good thing I could do, playing the songs for my dear grandchild.'

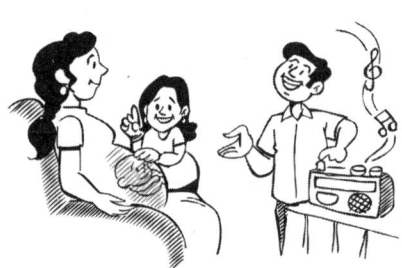

Tripura's father plays the baby a song. Tripura's sister talking to the baby

'No Dad, you are doing the best things for your grandchild and the baby knows and feels it. Whenever you are around, the baby feels your presence and enjoys it very much.'

'Do you think so?'

'Yes, Dad, I know for sure!'

Tripura's father plays Shiva Stotram for the baby and the baby again responds. Tripura and her baby rejoice in the journey of pregnancy together along with her family.

It is night-time and Tripura receives a phone call from her husband because she is staying at her mother's house for her delivery and he is at his house.

'Tripu, how are you dear, how's our baby doing?'

'We are both doing great. Honey! I am so happy that you have agreed to my request and keep your promise to call every night on the phone, and talk to me and, more importantly, to our baby. I know you are very busy and you must definitely be very tired after work. But you are calling me despite that. I am so touched by your love and affection!'

'What are you saying, Tripu? You are carrying our first baby and Mother Nature has been so kind to bless us with this baby. I am busy at work, but this is my life. Talking to you and our baby is the happiest moment of my life. I miss you both during the day and only after talking to you both do I feel relaxed. I sleep well only after our phone call every night. Let me talk to our baby.'

'Sure, dear.'

'Hi, sweetheart, this is Dad here. I think you have started identifying me through my voice now. How are you doing? Had your dinner? Did you listen to your favourite Shiva Stotram today? And did you dance to your favourite film song? My dear baby, I am so happy that you are surrounded by loving hearts. To all of us, you mean the most! Be happy, grow well and please stay in your mother's womb for nine months, safe and strong. Till then, we will all be in close touch with you. Dad will call you every night and I will try to visit you in person on some weekends. Oh, are you listening? I can feel it! Okay, dear, it's time for you and Mom to go to bed and sleep well. I will call again tomorrow night at the same time. Love you both, Mom and baby! Sleep well, Tripu, sweet dreams!' 'Sweet dreams to you, too!'

Right from the fifth month of Tripura's pregnancy, her mother used to count the movements of the baby, by keeping her hand on the abdomen. Her mother observed that for every specific number count, there was specific movement count from the baby. Tripura's mother kept this truth to herself and she kept track of the baby's well-being in her daughter's womb by regularly checking the baby's movement counts. Tripura did her part by properly talking to her baby.

An interesting observation

One morning, in the ninth month, Tripura's mother said the baby's movement had slowed down, but Tripura shot back that everything was fine. But in the evening, Tripura complained of decrease in the baby's movement, and they rushed to the hospital. After checking the heartbeat and looking at the ultrasound scan, the baby was found to be normal. Tripura was given IV fluid and, after some time, her mom kept her hands on her daughter's abdomen and declared that the baby was fine. Only after some time was Tripura able to confirm it. I understood the heightened sensitivity of the baby in the womb. The delivery was normal and safe. Tripura delivered a healthy baby boy and his

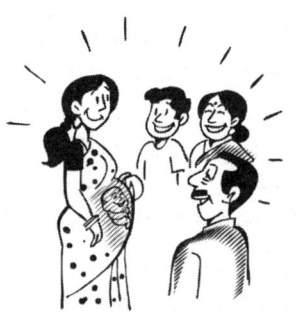

The elder child, grandmother, family and friends talking to the baby

family named him Akhilesh. The baby bonded very well with his grandparents and Indhu. When his grandfather crooned the first two or three lines of the film song that Akhilesh used to enjoy when he was in the womb, he became very happy and smiled. He would respond with continuous 'Hmm . . . Hmm' when his grandfather picked him up. That was his way of pleading with his grandfather to talk to him and play songs and chants for him. Akilesh would also answer with his eyes whenever people close to him talked to him. He was friendly and smiled even at strangers who came to see him. If he felt uncomfortable, he cried a little. So wonderful is the world of babies!

In the words of a jubilant Tripura, 'All thanks to Dr Andal, who gave us the wonderful tool of Talking to the Baby in the Womb. It is because of talking to the baby that we are on cloud nine with my very happy son, Akhilesh!'

That's the story of Tirpura. Anybody, be it the older child, grandmother, family or friends can sing for the baby in the womb and they will see that the baby bonds well with them after birth.

It is interesting to know the impact of music on Albert Einstein, the greatest scientist of the twentieth century. A little-known fact about Einstein is that when he was young, he did extremely poorly in school. His teachers told his parents to take him out of school because he was 'too stupid to learn' and it would be a waste of resources for the school to invest time and energy in his education. Albert's parents bought him a violin. Albert became good at the violin. Music was the key that helped Albert become one of the smartest men who ever lived. Einstein himself says that the reason for his smartness was because he played the violin. He loved the music of Mozart and Bach the most. A friend of Einstein, G.J. Withrow, revealed that Einstein figured out his problem and the equations by improvising on the violin.

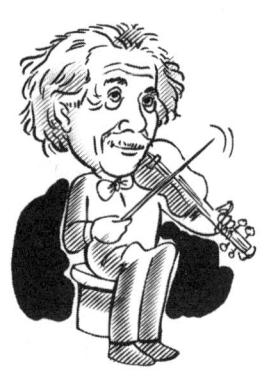

Albert Einstein, the violin is the sharpener of his intelligence.

Says Dr Verny, 'A four-or five-month-old fetus definitely responds to sound and melody - and responds in very discriminating ways. Put Vivaldi on a phonograph and even the most agitated baby relaxes. Put Beethoven on and even the calmest child starts kicking and moving. Soft, soothing voice makes him feel loved and wanted He is mature enough intellectually to sense the emotional tone of the maternal voice.'[*]

Effects of Music

These effects are instant and long-lasting. Music is supposed to link all the emotional, spiritual and physical

---

[*] Verny with Kelly. *Secret Life*, p. 21).

elements of the universe. Music can also be used to change a person's mood, and has been found to cause physical responses in many people simultaneously.

On Body

It decreases blood pressure and enhances the ability to learn. Music affects the amplitude and frequency of brain waves, which can be measured by an electro-encephalogram. Music also affects the breathing rate and electrical resistance of the skin.

On Mind

As the body becomes relaxed, the mind is able to concentrate more easily. The simultaneous left and right brain action maximizes learning and retention of information. Students' listening skills also improved through music education. Musical training has an effect on how the brain gets wired for general cognitive functioning related to memory and attention. It is clear that music is good for children's cognitive development and that music should be part of the preschool and primary school curriculum. It helps in improving learning and neuroplasticity, which is the brain's ability to repair connections and form new neural connections (wiring) in response to a new situation. A study of the brains of musicians shows more than five times as many interconnections in the brain as in non-musicians. Student musicians have an average of eleven IQ points higher than non-musicians.

On Relationship

Music enhances prenatal bonding. One of the most intimate and pleasurable events experienced by the baby in the womb is his mother's singing. It is also one of the first dialogues exchanged between mother and child. Songs that communicate love, acceptance, and welcome are most reassuring to the baby. This is a two-way process whereby the mother and child form a close attachment, developing trust, a feeling of safety and a sense of belonging. All other relationships will depend on the quality of this first exchange. If we are nurtured lovingly with consistency, then we will most likely treat others in the same manner.

Music Therapy

Music and sound are beginning to play an active role in medicine as evidenced by studies in neurobiology and psychology. In this regard, music therapy is also making a contribution to the healing arts.

Scientific Evidence

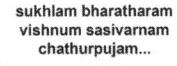

Dr Suzanne Hanser, Berklee's Music Therapy Department chair, says, 'There is scientific evidence that music therapy

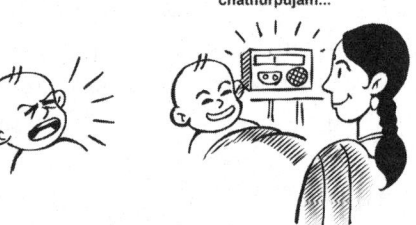

influences the children on the autism spectrum in several ways, like enhancing skills in communication, interpersonal relationships, self-regulation, coping strategies, stress management, and focusing attention.'[*]

According to a UK study, children recognize and prefer music they were exposed to in the womb for at least a year after they are born. The study by Dr Alexandra Lamont from the music research group at the university's School of Psychology confirms the same.[†]

Let us see some real-life examples:

'Hello, Nithya! How's the baby doing?'

'Yes, Doctor, all okay except that every evening at 5 p.m., the baby feels very uncomfortable and starts crying at a high pitch. However much we all try to stop his crying, he feels restless in the evenings.' 'Did you see a paediatrician?'

'Yes, ma'am. He said everything is fine.'

'Hmmm. Well, during your pregnancy, did you do anything specifically in the evening that you have discontinued after the delivery?'

'To be honest, I discontinued doing many things that I used to do when I was pregnant, Doctor.'

'No, that's not what I meant. What did you do around 5 p.m. during your pregnancy? Try to recollect. After all, it was not that long ago. You must have had a routine during your pregnancy.'

'Oh, yes, Doctor, during the pregnancy, every evening at 5 p.m., I used to listen to Vishnu Sahasranamam, but

---

[*] Burg, Liz. 'Music Therapy in Autism for Families and Professionals', Berklee College of Music, https://college.berklee.edu/news/3726/music-therapy-in-autism-for-families-and-profess, accessed on 21 August 2025.

[†] Lamont, Alexandra, and Hargreaves, David. *The Psychology of Musical Development* (London: Cambridge University Press, 2017).

after delivery, I stopped doing so, not deliberately, but because of visitors and the baby's feeding schedules.'

'Please continue the practice and tell me how the baby responds. Call me after three days, Nithya.'

Three days went by and I received a call from Nithya; her voice was filled with happiness and relief. She said, 'Doctor, I really don't know how to thank you! My baby has stopped crying completely! All that my husband and I did was resume the practice of playing Vishnu Sahasranamam in the same volume as before. My baby would calm down immediately and within minutes, enjoy the chant. He connects with the Sahasranamam totally and feels at ease and he is very happy. Oh doctor, what a feeling it is! You are an ace at the language spoken by babies! A million thanks to you, Doctor!'

'Nithya, keep playing Vishnu Sahasranamam to your child till he grows big and chants himself. His speech, language skills, IQ and happiness all increase by listening to his womb song. This would be the best gift you can give to your child next to breast milk.'

'Sure, ma'am. I'll follow your advice.'

When the boy was three years of age, he started chanting Vishnu Sahasranamam to everybody's pleasant surprise. Sirisha touched my heart with words of wisdom. She said that the baby responded to the chant and smiled at her on hearing the chants of Om Nama Shivaya and slept peacefully. She used to listen to the chant during her pregnancy at night. Whenever she talked to the baby, he responded with his eyes. When called by name, he turned his head. And when asked to stop crying, he stopped immediately. This is the result of the strong intention of Sirisha to bond with the baby right from the period of pregnancy.

Monica was pregnant. She felt that the baby had stopped moving. She got scared, and during her consultation she said the previous day she had been listening to peppy numbers of a famous actor. The baby had started moving vigorously in the womb as if it was dancing along with the hyped-up number.

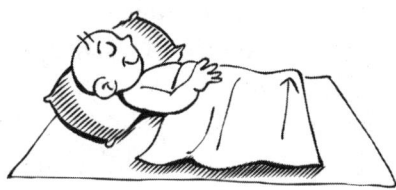

Om Namashivaya chant acted like a lullaby.

Monica had felt extremely uncomfortable and hence had scolded the baby and had asked it to stop dancing to the song. After this incident, she could not appreciate the baby's movements. Then, on doctor's suggestions, Monica apologized to the baby and asked the baby to move again and, after some time, she felt the movement. Next time, when another peppy number of the same actor started playing, Monica requested the baby to enjoy the song and dance gently and this time the baby moved to the song happily but the movements were not vigorous. So sensitive and cooperative the babies are!

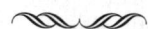

Rajeshwari is a very good singer. When she became pregnant, she used to sing and listen to Annamayya

Keerthans. After delivery, when the baby was just two months old, she found to her surprise that her daughter hummed the raga along with her. More amazing was the fact that during the feeding, whenever there was any disturbance, the baby used to prompt her mother with a very clear 'Amma'. First, Rajeshwari thought that it was a rare sound accidentally made by her baby. But in due course, she found that her baby was clearly calling her 'Amma'. Then, she remembered that while Talking to the Baby in her Womb, she used to tell the baby to be a very good linguist and that she should learn languages fast along with music. The baby took the cue and started pronouncing the sweetest word 'Amma' so early. She starting speaking early and liked womb songs. As she grew up, she learnt Telugu and English very well, and from a young age took part in competitions and bagged prizes.

Chitra was an ardent admirer of Annamacharya and was listening to his Keerthanas during pregnancy. When her son was three, he started singing Annamaya songs. At the age of seven, he learnt to play the keyboard without anyone teaching him. That was the impact of exposure during pregnancy.

The Don'ts

If you're listening to music for prolonged periods, it is best to keep the volume below 50dB, the usual sound level maintained in most neonatal intensive care units. It is not a good idea to use headphones on your belly since the music is up close and may overstimulate the baby. Another important point is that the music bypasses the mother and goes directly to the baby. It may confuse the baby and the required response will not be there.

An obsessive need to create a musical genius might cause you to push hard and set a standard that your child may never meet.

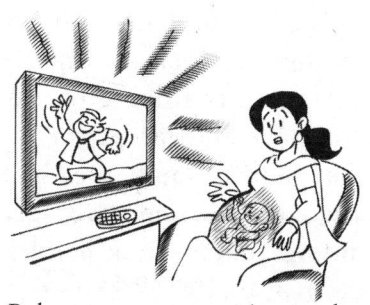

Baby starts to move vigorously after listening to a fast-beat song

Such stress occurs only when the mother focuses on the outcome, and holds the baby responsible without developing a strong bond. There will be results no doubt, but they will not be remarkable. It is like a song pleasant to the ears but not a solace for the soul. There may be stress for both the mother and the baby. This is the way of managing moms (only

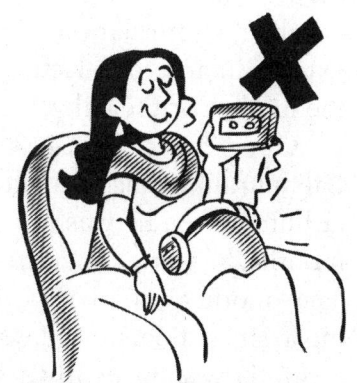

Don't keep headphones over mom's belly, as it confuses the baby

having; being = personality, having = achievement). 'Having' has a limited bandwidth.

When being is added to it, the bandwidth becomes unlimited, yielding spectacular results.

Managing moms = weak bonding + affirmations done mechanically + belief = expected result (achievement). It may be pleasant to the ears, but not a solace to the soul; sometimes causing stress to the mother as well as the baby. When a recording, affirmation (Talking to the Baby) suggestion is done with love and care, strong bonding is created between the mother and the baby. When Personality is strengthened, the baby gets totally aligned with the mother, understands her desires and is able to fulfil her desires easily. When personality is strengthened, excellence (achievement and skills) is a natural offshoot. Wonderful effects are possible. It just happens. This is the way of nurturing moms. Nurturing moms = strong bonding + affirmations with love and care + belief = extraordinary, long-lasting results. No stress to either the mother or the baby.

Our great music maestro, the late M. Balamuralikrishna recalled how his mother used to sing at home when he was in her womb. At the age of two months, he started saying syllables and later humming. The mother of the popular musician, Bombay Jayasree recalls how she ardently desired the baby she was carrying to become a great musician. In both these instances, the mothers are nurturers and their intention was strong, so their wish was fulfilled.

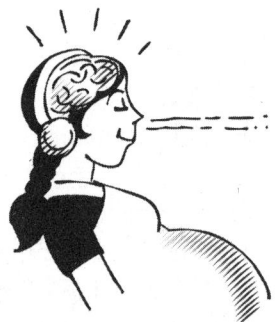

Mom enjoys the music

A child is able to remember the 'womb song' after it is delivered. We ask the mother to select a song which she enjoys. It is a common observation that the baby also enjoys it, remembers it after it comes out.

Benefits of Listening to Music for the Mother

- It improves the bonding between the mother and the baby.
- She is able to come out of stress and overcome the physical ailments or complications, if any, and handle pregnancy confidently.
- Makes the mother relaxed and helps her feel less pain during labour, aiding in normal delivery.

Benefits of Listening to Music for the Baby after Delivery

- Womb song is like a lullaby, makes a crying baby stop and puts it to sleep.
- Helps in taking breastfeeding better.
- There is heightened awareness in these babies after birth and they smile and talk early and easily.

Listening to music if continued after delivery, helps babies talk early and have superior language skills. It also improves mathematical and communication skills. The heartbeat of the mother is the first familiar rhythm for the baby. Heartbeat plays a major part in reassurance and, as per Dr Verny, it acts as a major life support system in the world of babies. Dr Verny terms a mother's heartbeat lovingly and rightfully as the 'womb music.'

That's why when the mother or anyone lulls the baby by placing it on the left side of the chest close to the heart, the baby hears again the familiar rhythm and calms down and falls asleep soon.

Lullaby, the bedtime song, is known by different names in different languages.

(Hindi: lori; Telugu: laalipaata; Kannada: Laalihaadu; Malayalam: tharattupattu; Tamil: Thalaatupaatu)

Regardless of the meaning of their words, lullabies are rooted in 'love, tenderness and caring' and have a peaceful, hypnotic quality, says Zoe Palmer, a musician working on a lullabies project at the Royal London Hospital. She has found that 'Wherever you go in the world, women use the same tones, the same sort of way of singing to their babies. Many lullabies are very basic. With just a few words repeated again and again, lullabies are remarkably similar across cultures.'

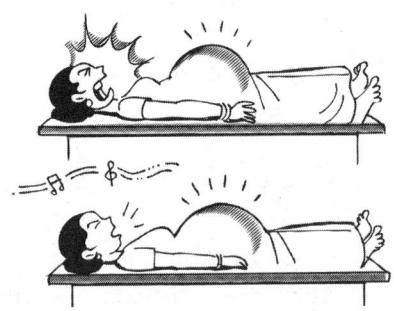

When she listens to the womb song, she is more relaxed and feels less pain during labour

Colwyn Trevarthen, professor of child psychology at the University of Edinburgh and vice-president of the British Association for Early Childhood Education, says, 'What's particularly astonishing is how precisely the baby responds—in coos and gestures—often exactly in time with the pulse and bar structure of her sounds. Baby and mother get into the groove.'*

Lullabies belong to the instinctive nature of motherhood.

Important Long-Term Use

Mothers should continue 'womb song' after delivery. Even two or three lines are enough. Slowly, the baby starts humming the tune. As the baby grows, they should be made to sing it daily. This conditions the baby to be happy. Whenever he/she is upset, the song immediately relaxes the mood and acts as a great stress buster. It also helps in improving health and hence it can be considered as a great lifelong gift to the baby.

Birth Song of Africa

There is a Himba Tribe in Africa where, when a woman decides that she will have a child, she goes off and sits under a tree, by herself; she can hear the song of the child that wants to

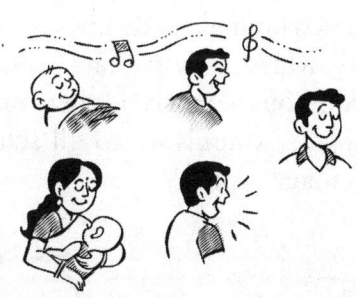

Music influences all stages and ages of life

---

* Perry, Nina. 'The Universal Language of Lullabies', BBC (21 January 2013), https://www.bbc.com/news/magazine-21035103, acessed on 22 August 2025.

come. And after she has heard the song of this child, she comes back to the child's father, teaches him, and then they sing the song of the child, as a way to invite it. When the mother is pregnant, the mother teaches that child's song to the midwives and the old women of the village, so that when the child is born, all sing the child's song to welcome it. And then, as the child grows up, the other villagers are taught the child's song, they sing it at marriages and other occasions till the end of life.

Let us see quotes of some famous personalities.

Dr Rob Hicks: 'Music rewards us in so many ways. At one end of the scale, music is energizing and at the other end, it can help to calm the most stressful situation.'

Napoleon understood the enormous power of music. He summed it up by saying, 'Give me control over he who shapes the music of a nation, and I care not who makes the laws'.

Maestro Ilaiyaraaja says, 'If you want to completely root out terrorism, then music education should be made compulsory to all schoolchildren in the five to ten age group.'

Boris Brott

Boris Brott is a Canadian conductor and motivational speaker. He is the conductor of the Hamilton, Ontario

Philharmonic Symphony. When an interviewer asked him how he had become interested in music, he answered, 'You know, this may sound strange, but music has been a part of me since before birth.'

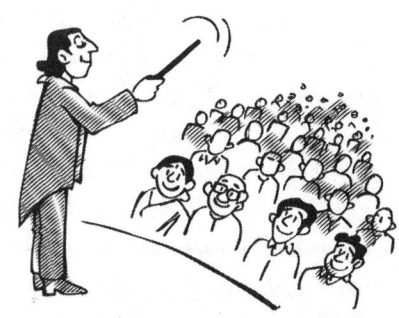

'Well,' said Brott, 'as a young man, I was mystified by this unusual ability I had to play certain pieces of sight unseen I'd be conducting a score for the first time and suddenly, the cello line would jump out at me; I'd know the flow of the piece even before I turned the page of the score. One day I mentioned this to my mother, who is a professional cellist. I thought she'd be intrigued because it was always the cello line that was so distinct in my mind. She was; but when she heard what the pieces were, the mystery solved itself quickly. All the scores I knew sight unseen were ones she had played while she was pregnant with me.'*

Sahana: As a doctor with many years of experience, do you recommend any specific raga, a song, mantra, chant, a CD or a music album that is particularly beneficial to a pregnant woman?'

---

* Verny with Kelly. *Secret Life*, pp. 22–23.

Doctor: 'No. I don't recommend anything to anyone. Because music influences people in different ways; what is soothing to one, may not appeal as much to the other. Thus, I leave it to mothers to choose their own music. It could be a mantra, shloka, a specific album, any raga or a movie song. The important thing is that a mother should enjoy the music and pass on the wonderful feeling to the baby. When the mother finds the music soothing, naturally it influences the baby positively. So, you can choose any music that makes you happy and relaxed.

Shankar: Thanks a lot for this wealth of information. It's indeed a feast for the mind and heart.

Doctor: Thanks Shankar and Sahana. It was a memorable experience; this sylvan setting provided the right ambience for the topic.

Sahana: Thanks a lot, Aunty. I've understood the influence of music in the womb. Can we also instil the spirit of sports during pregnancy?

Doctor: Yes. Sahana. I'll talk about it in next session. Bye! Regards to your Mom.

Sahana: Okay. Bye, Aunty!

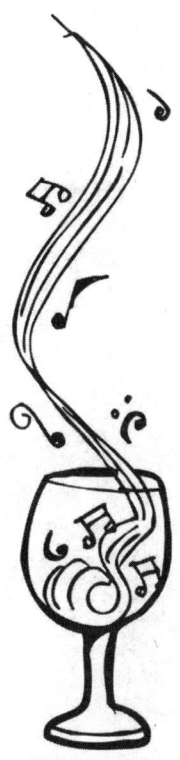

If you pour music into whatever's wrong,
it's sure to help you out.

7

Sports

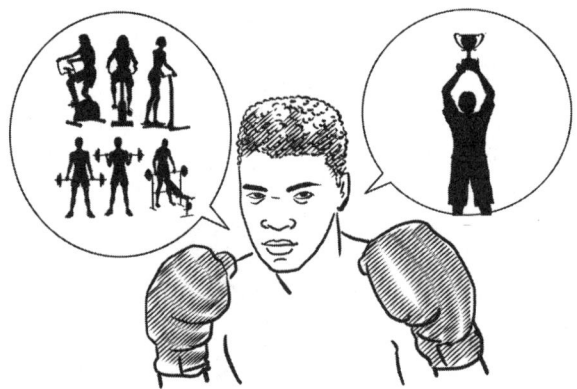

Champions are not made in gyms. They are made from a desire, dream and a vision.

—Muhammad Ali,
heavy-weight champion

Sahana: Aunty, Mummy has come to meet you.
Doctor: Wow! Vijaya! It's been long time since we met. What a pleasant surprise!
Vijaya: Hello, Andal! It's indeed a happy moment for me. I'm seeing you after a long time. One quiz for you, dear.
Doctor: Thank you so much, Vijaya. I'm eager to know your question. Let me see if I can pass your test.
Vijaya: I have brought a home-made goodie for you. My mom made it specially for you. Can you guess?
Doctor: Is it the yummy kammarkat (coconut and jaggery burfi), Aunty used to make when we were in school?
Vijaya: Yes! You are right. Glad you remember it.
Doctor: How can we forget the good old times?
They all relax, eating snacks and reminiscing about old times.
Sahana: Aunty, my friend Rati loves sports, and she aspired to become a tennis player but couldn't go beyond the school level. Is there a way that she can give birth to a sporting champion through the Talking to the Baby in the Womb technique? Does it sound overambitious? Or acting like a managing mother?'
Doctor: No, not at all. It is perfectly normal to dream about having a sporting champion. Why not? One can raise a sports star inside the womb by effectively doing Talking to the Baby in the Womb. You need to build the spirit without being pushy. Become a nurturing mom, build rapport with the baby and then share your dreams. Let me share the details of how Lochana

gave birth to a champion cricketer by effectively using Talking to the Baby in the Womb.

'My dear brother, this *teeka* is for you. I went to the temple and prayed for your big win once again!'

'Thank you, Preethi, it means a lot to me.'

'Hey Sujeeth, this is for you, light-weight gloves and pads.' 'Wow, Dad, I didn't expect this.'

'Yes, you didn't, but I noticed that you needed light-weight accessories to perform better.'

'Thank you, Dad, I can't thank you enough for this wonderful gift!'

'Sujeeth, come here for a minute.'

'Yes, Grandma.'

'Here's your curd and sugar blessing. Show your hand, this holy thread is for your safety as well as success!'

'Bless me, Grandma. Your blessing is always the best assurance of my success.'

Sujeeth touches the feet of his loving grandmother and she blesses him with a heart full of love and affection. Preethi enters the kitchen and sees her mom, Lochana, quietly arranging the breakfast plates. Preethi goes near her mom and talks.

'Mom, what are you doing here? There, Dad and Grandma are wishing Sujeet all the very best. I can see Dad living on the edge on the days when Sujeet plays cricket matches. He will soon be selected to play in the national team for the country. I can only smile imagining Dad's plight then. Grandma starts chanting and carries on her all-day prayers. I am edgy in my own ways because I want my brother to score the highest and win the Man of the Match title in every match he plays. But you, on the other hand, are never tensed. You are sort of so sure about the victory graph of Sujeet. What is the secret behind your relaxed stature, my dear mom?'

Sujeet's father giving him gloves and his grandmother ties the scared thread on him.

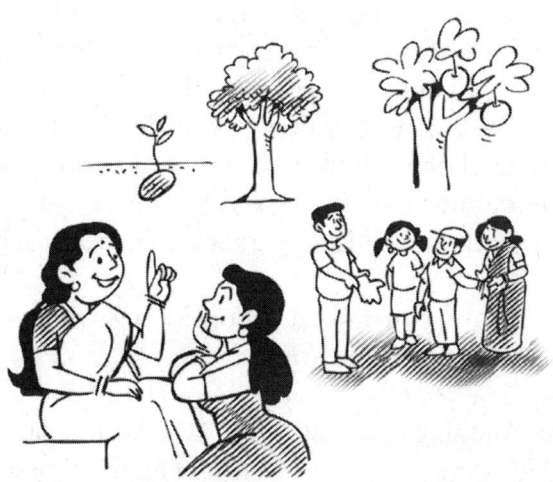

Mom says that she sure is sure of Surjeet's victory because she knew the seed has been sown.

'Preethi, let us help your brother leave for his match first. We will settle down to talk about this interesting question of yours. Deal?'
    'Deal, Mom'
'Set the plates on the table first.'
    'Done!'

Sujeet finishes breakfast, and as he starts, he comes near his mom and with a loving smile, touches her feet. Lochana, stops him midway, hugs him and tells him in a calm and clear voice. 'Just keep your eye on the ball, the victory is yours as usual. You are born to win big and remember this often and always!'

'Thank you, Mom! Your words give me all the charge that I need to win; it works like a mantra!'

Sujeet leaves. Lochana's husband gets busy with his work. Grandma begins her prayer routine in her room. Once the house gets calm, Lochana and Preethi finish their breakfast and settle down on the sofa to chat about the most interesting question extended by Preethi.

'Now, tell me, Mom. How can you be so calm and confident about Sujeet's cricketing career?'

'It is because I did my part when Sujeet was in my womb.'

'What are you talking about? How can you do your part before his birth?'

'Yes. I talked to him as per the advice of our beloved Doctor Andal. I talked to you too. Well, you know your dad is mad about cricket. I wanted my first baby to be a talented cricketer bringing laurels to the nation. I wanted him to be the best gift I offer to your dad.'

'Oh, I didn't know about this "gift concept" so far. It's great! What did you do to talk to your "Gift"?'

'First, I thanked God for giving him to me. I loved him so much and I wanted him to understand and accept me. I could feel the response. I shared my likes, dislikes, dreams, just like sharing them with a friend. We enjoyed each other's company. Even now Sujeet understands my feelings better than your dad in some issues.'

'Yes! I've noticed it, Ma.'

'I spoke a lot about cricket and I watched a lot of cricket matches when I was pregnant with Sujeet. I told him, he too would love cricket like your dad, enjoy playing the game, feel at ease and be focused on regular practice and test matches. He, too, would become a great cricket star. Slowly, I started feeling confident that my baby was created to bloom as a wonderful cricketer.

When Sujeet was born and as he showed a keen interest in the game of cricket, I knew that Talking to the Baby in the Womb had started showing signs of its magic. So, I registered him for the best coaching classes. He has so far not missed a single coaching session. He says cricket is his life and that's his dedication. I know the seed I'd sown. I see the plant and leaves. So, I am sure about the fruit. That's why I am not excited or tense about his matches. He is born to win.'

'Oh super! Now I know the secret behind your cool demeanour. What did you talk to me about?'

'Yes, I told you to choose the field of your interest and do well in that. I wanted to give you the freedom of selecting the field. But I knew that you would choose some form of art. See how well you are doing today as an artist! Your art has started earning recognition!'

'All thanks to Doctor Andal and her Talking to the Baby in the Womb technique!'

Lochana's husband switches on the television and they all happily settle down to watch Sujeet's match.

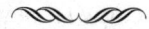

Let us see some real-life sports persons' stories.

Jennifer Capriati is a famous, much-loved tennis star. Family legend holds that Jennifer began playing tennis while still in the womb. Approximately seventeen hours before her birth, Stefano had taken Denise out to play tennis. 'He knew she would be a tennis player even before she was born,' her mother later said. Jennifer was a precociously gifted athlete from the time she was an infant. She learned to swim before she learned to crawl and was able to swing all the way across a set of monkey bars before she could walk.

Google still holds record of the miracle called **Martha Bissah** and celebrates her as follows.

Martha Bissah: A nearly aborted foetus is now a world champion, seventeen-year-old Martha Bissah, tells the inspiring story of how her mother, who was an athlete and a footballer in her school days, was in a dilemma to either abort a one-month-old pregnancy for greener pastures abroad, or to keep the baby and choose to endure the hustles of life in her third-world country, Ghana. But for reasons that one may not easily comprehend, the selfless teen mother, who was seventeen years old at the time, abandoned her dreams and made what some would call a stupid or weird decision by insisting she would keep the baby. She thus forfeited that rare opportunity.

Now, call it a miracle or destiny, the foetus, which was not aborted in exchange for stardom and perhaps money in women's football, has supernaturally turned out to become a world champion in athletics, inexplicably also at the age of seventeen.

You can interpret it whichever way you wish, but the bottom line remains that this is undoubtedly a moving story that carries a lesson for all, especially for those who will easily opt for abortions in similar or isolated circumstances. It is often noticed that when a talented mother or father did not find an opportunity to express their talents to the fullest and they still nurture their baby in the womb with all care and love, it is assured that the baby thus born achieves highest ranks in the field in which the parent couldn't succeed. This brings about the fact of epigenetics that with environment, genes bloom to settle the unuttered desires of the parents. So intelligent are the foetuses.

Mohammed Ali's daughter, **Laila Ali,** is the super middle-weight champion, and was unbeaten till 2014 with twenty-four wins, no losses, no draws. Similar in the case of Bruce Lee and his son **Brandon lee**. It is noted that the offspring chose the same field as their fathers did, becoming champions in the same sport. This can be attributed to the fact that the wives of these legends get inspired by their husbands, watch their husbands in action during their pregnancy days and secretly hail, admire and love the success of their husbands. This leads them to dream of their babies in their wombs as worthy successors of their legendary spouses. 'It is in the blood,' as they say. When their champion fathers talk to their wives, the babies listen and when they are personally talked to by their dads, they take the cue and develop a keen interest in their 'family sport'. Nature, the genes, and nurture, the grooming, play a major part in carrying the legacy of family sports like a relay game.

We can also see that the dreams of some of the close family members also come true.

Rafael Nadal, the ace tennis champion, is coached by his own uncle, who dreamt of his nephew making it big in the game of tennis. The same is the case with women's tennis champion, Maria Sharapova. Her dad's biggest dream of making his daughter a grand star of tennis and all his efforts of moving to America for the same cause have brought the sweetest fruits for him today.

Susheela, the mother of Grand Master **Vishwanathan Anand**, sculpted him into what he is today. Anand would watch his mother and sister play chess and that's how he got interested in chess. But the truth is, Anand's mother used to be a great chess player right from her young days. Naturally, she wished her baby to be a grand player in the game of chess. She has just created a better version of her talent by nurturing the baby's personality with love and care before and after birth, like her finding of the TAL Chess Club for Anand to get groomed as a master ace chess champion. As per the report, Mr Subbaraman from Chennai gave up his job to help his daughters Vijayalakshmi, Meenakshi and Bhanupriya follow their chess careers. Vijayalakshmi and Meenakshi are women's grand masters now.

Babies in the womb are sensitive and sensible beyond our perceptions. So, make the baby in the womb feel wanted and loved both from the conscious and subconscious levels. The aim of Talking to the Baby in the Womb is just to bond with the baby, make rapport and enjoy the companionship. (being = personality; having = achievement and skills). Skills have a limited bandwidth. When personality is added to it, the bandwidth becomes unlimited, yielding spectacular results. When a recording of a suggestion is done with love and care, it creates a strong bond between mother and baby. When personality is thus strengthened, the baby gets totally aligned with the mother, understands her desires and is able to fulfil her desires easily. When personality is strengthened, excellence and skills are a natural off-shoot and wonderful and miraculous results are possible.

It just happens. There is no stress for mother and baby. This is the way of nurturing moms. Nurturing Moms = strong bonding + affirmations with love and care + belief = extraordinary and long-lasting results (personality + skills). When we are happy, positive beliefs get deeply and easily imprinted in the subconscious mind. The effect of affirmations coming out of strong bonding is like the mesmerizing effect of the captivating music of a great master totally immersed in it. If the recording is perfect with love, the execution and the expression is effortless, easy and of unimaginably high quality. Excellence in any field can be easily achieved. The intensity of the mother's feeling and the belief are the prime factors that make the recording effective and long-lasting. This is the way of nurturing moms. If, for some reason, the mother is unable to talk, she can play the songs that would let the baby know about her desires. She can express her desires to the closest person to her and let that person talk to the baby. Let the husband also tell the baby that the world is waiting to applaud its achievements.

What Not to Do

Keep one important thing in mind—don't put pressure on the baby by forcing or ordering it. Your baby can be your dream-come-true, but it is not your robot. Respect your baby by giving it the blueprint of your beautiful dreams to work out and build on. Never assume that your baby is obliged to live out every dream of yours that you yourself could not fulfil. Your baby has you as the channel to enter the world. But it is not your shadow. While as a mother, your health and life are of prime importance, as a proud co-creator, you should respect your baby as an individual life towards which you have a great responsibility.

When the bond is not strong, the recording becomes mechanical, the mother focuses only on the outcome, and holds the baby responsible. It is like a song pleasant to the ears, but doesn't give any solace to the soul. Sometimes, there may be stress for both the mother and the baby. This is the way of managing moms. Managing Moms = weak bonding + mechanical affirmations + belief = expected results (Only having skills). Stress may be there for both the mother and the baby.

Abhimanyu

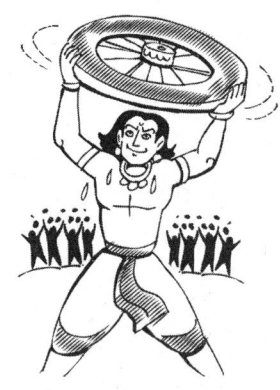

Abhimanyu entering the Chakravyuka

Abhimanyu was the son of Arjuna and Subhadra. He was very skilled at archery and was the pride of the Pandavas. Even as a lad, Abhimanyu was very strong and brave. While Abhimanyu was in his mother's womb, he heard Arjuna telling

Subhadra how to fend off warriors when they surround you in a Chakravyuha or intricate maze during a battle. Arjuna explained to Subhadra how to enter a Chakravyuha, but before he could explain how to get out of it he was called away. But whatever he had heard Arjuna say, Abhimanyu carefully stored it in his memory. He grew up to be a brave, handsome young man. Many years later, during the Mahabharata war at Kurukshetra, the Kauravas set up a Chakravyuha and challenged the Pandavas to come forward and break it. However, only Arjuna, who was fighting elsewhere, knew the technique of doing so. At that stage, to save the honour of the Pandavas, Abhimanyu came forward and offered his services for the task of breaking the Chakravyuha. Despite his incomplete knowledge of the technique, he entered the grid and overcame one circle after another and fought valiantly. Abhimanyu had listened to Arjun's talk with such rapt attention that he could remember the details even after so many years.

Recent scientific findings have shown that babies can indeed hear and learn when still inside their mother's womb.

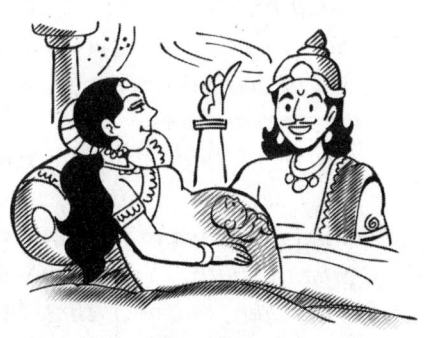

Arjun telling Shubadra, when she was carrying Abhimanyu, about the secrets of entering the Chakravyuka

Sahana: Thank you, Aunty, for sharing such inspiring stories. Is there anything that you want to add?

Doctor: Sahana, some parents provide necessary moral and material support to help the kids realize their dreams themselves. These are parents who prepare the children for the journey on any road. Another type of parent prepares the road for the children without paying attention to preparing them. You can raise a champion by instilling positive values about being competitive and winning through fair means.

Sahana: Aunty, what sort of exercise do you advise during pregnancy; should I practice prenatal yoga?

Doctor: Sahana, I tell the mothers to remember that pregnancy is a natural function of the body and not a disease, even if they go to the doctor and take medicines (of course, mostly supplements of iron, calcium, etc.). Research shows that pregnant mothers can do the work they were doing before pregnancy. We advise bed rest only in cases of previous abortions or miscarriages, twins, polyhydramnios (excess of amniotic fluid in the uterus), etc.

I see two groups of mothers, one that follows the Vinayaka Swami path and the other the Subrahmanya Swami path. You remember? To get the mango, Vinayaka believed that his parents represented the world, and so went round them. Subramanya circled the world in his peacock vaahana *(vehicle). Similarly, one group of mothers believe that pregnancy is natural, and their mothers did only household work and had normal deliveries. For them, doing household work is the sure and time-tested way of physical preparation for delivery. The modern, tech-savvy group of mothers feel they need to know everything about pregnancy and delivery from a Google guru, follow diet and exercise scrupulously and feel satisfied that they have taken utmost care for the baby. These mothers do prenatal yoga under the guidance of a trainer. That also gives good results. Both groups are on the right path. They get the desired results if they do it regularly with interest and conviction. We must remember that more than the effort, the intention and belief do not have the final say in getting the result. It is because the function of delivery is controlled by hormones that are dependent on emotions.*

I advise mothers to be active, perform routine household work, and do walking and breathing exercises from the beginning. If doing it from the fag end of the eighth month or the beginning of the ninth month, it would be advisable for them to do a few more exercises such as squatting, butterfly, kegel and climbing up the steps. I advise them to do the exercises with interest so as to make them effective. The support of the husband or any other member of the family will go a long way in achieving the desired results. Remember, our elders did only household work. The mental preparation (moral support of the elders), along with this type of physical preparation, helped in their having an easy, normal delivery, before the era of hospital delivery. It is not only the household work, but also the positive mindset and moral support that yielded better results.

Vijaya: Andal, I want to know something about exercise. This is for my personal interest and may therefore be out of context.

Doctor: Please feel free to ask.

Vijaya: I only do household work. Not used to going to the gym. I feel guilty about it; any easy suggestions for me?

Doctor: Vijaya, don't worry. I'll tell you, your household work is a 'care-giving activity'. It's both self-care and family care! You should be proud that you are both a home-maker and an educationist. Explore an activity that interests you. Do it regularly. This will keep you physically and mentally fit. Planning, doing with interest and consistency are the key factors here.

Nandi, gastroenterologist from the US, says: 'We can become health heroes by understanding the purpose and following suitable food habits and activity with interest and passion. That way, our mental and physical health will be good like that of our forefathers.

A health hero knows why he or she is exercising. Knowing the reason for the activity will help motivation and dedication, ensuring success. Movement is for increased well-being, to achieve health, not just beautifully sculpted bodies and not to conform to the temporary standards of society. You don't have to be an Olympic athlete or have the quickness, strength, or grace of your heroes. You simply have to find the desire and the heart.

Everything you do is an opportunity to burn calories, and every object around you is a potential weight to lift or ball to throw. Sidewalks are for walking, so do so as often as possible. Beat that batter by hand instead of using the mixer. Instead of taking the elevator, take the stairs. Park as far away from the entrance of the store as you can. Carry your own groceries. Do gardening in the yard. If you sit all day, stand up every hour and walk, stretch and breathe deeply for at least five minutes.

What you will get are the benefits of movement with purpose: weight control, increased energy, and improvement in your numbers, which gauge blood pressure, blood sugar levels, and cholesterol. The movement of the health hero can indeed heal the body and the mind. In fact, exercise can be as effective as some antidepressants in treating mild to moderate depression! 'Life is your workout, and it's free and you will always have time for it, unlike the three hours it takes to get in and out of a gym.' Once you find your favourite activity, do it regularly with interest.

Vijaya: Andal, you made my day through words of wisdom. I also learnt how I can support Sahana in her pregnancy.

Sahana: I need your advice on how to handle the issue of my vomiting.

Doctor: Good that you asked for help. In pregnancy, you should say goodbye to shyness, guilt and inhibition.

Vijaya: Andal, can I help Sahana with this vomiting? Poor thing! She is suffering a lot.

Doctor: Yes, Vijaya. You and Sahana can do a lot in this regard. Let me share my experiences about how elders can reassure an expecting mother.

F.A.I.L. means First Attempt Learning

E.N.D. means Effort Never Dies

N.O. means Next Opportunity

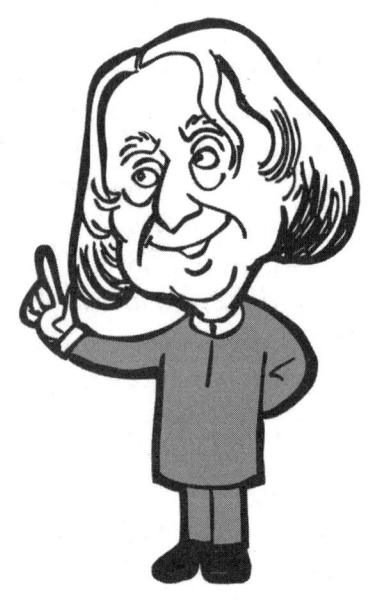

8

Happy Helpers in Reducing Nausea and Vomiting

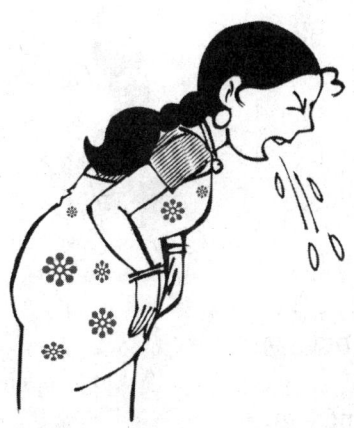

Positive thoughts may be the ultimate health tip
for a pregnant woman.

Sahana: Though I am confident now, what should I do when the vomiting becomes severe, Aunty?

Doctor: 'Don't worry. It is quite easy to handle vomiting if you are well informed and prepared.'

Vijaya: Andal, the problem is that when Sahana vomits, I get panicky. Only my mother is unruffled. She says casually that it's normal and will subside in a few months. I can't be cool like her.

Doctor: Yes, Vijaya, she is absolutely right. To make you understand the truth, let me share with you the story of Sheela.

'Why are you looking very tired and sad? Is there anything that I can do to cheer you up, Sheela dear?'

'No, Padma, this is one situation I have to bear alone. You are so sweet, but you can't help me.'

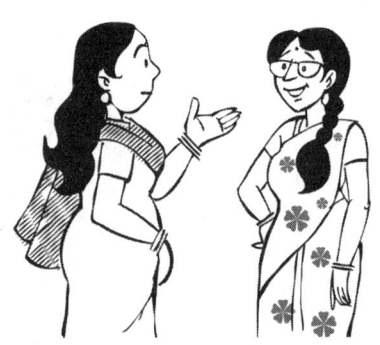

Asking for suggestions

'Try telling me. Maybe I can understand the problem. I am a senior when it comes to pregnancy, with a lot more experience. Sometimes just unburdening will provide a lot of relief.'

'It's my nausea and vomiting. Even medicines are not of much use in my case. Now you know that you cannot help me, right?'

'Maybe not directly, but I can help. More so, there is really someone who can directly help you!'

'Do you mean my doctor?'

'No, not your doctor, I meant your baby!'

'What are you saying? Are you joking?'

'Would I joke about this plight of yours? I mean what I say because I speak from first-hand experience!'

'Is that so?!'

'Yes, it is. If I narrate to you my experience with my daughter when I was carrying, then it will dawn on you.'

'Tell me, please. I am all ears for anything that would throw light on my vomiting.'

'When I became pregnant, I started throwing up, I mean I started vomiting. It was really bad; unbearable! I went to my gynaecologist for help.'

'Doctor, please do something. I have been having very severe and prolonged vomiting. I am not getting relief with the treatment. It's my fifth month of pregnancy and the vomiting is so severe. I am frequently on IV fluids (drips). I feel helpless about it. I want this baby to be safe and healthy. Is it possible?'

Doctor, 'I understand, Padma, try not to panic about this situation. I have successfully treated many cases like yours. I know about it very well. You need to do the following:

1. Changes in diet.
2. Take medicines regularly.
3. The most important one is that your worry and anxiety must be replaced by a secure feeling and peace of mind.

A useful tool in such a situation is Talking to the Baby in the Womb. Talk to your baby and ask for help. Your baby will help you. Your mom can help you in this as well. As she has already delivered you and your brother, her experience will help understand the point better.

Padma asks her mom, 'Ma, what will I ever do to *save* my baby?'

'Padma, stop crying! This despair, fear and depression are not good for your health. Try talking to your baby to create a possible, positive situation!'

'Ma, are you making fun of me? Dr Andal too suggested the same thing. But I thought she wanted to comfort me and that's why she suggested that playfully.'

'Certainly not, my darling; nobody knows better than Dr Andal about this. She has instructed me as to how to go about this and how to handle this. Nobody jokes in matters such as these. Your baby is my grandchild and I feel as protective about my child and the child inside my child! In fact, it's doubly protective that I feel! That's why I am suggesting the only effective way to help yourself and your child!'

'I still don't understand what you are trying to tell me, Ma . . .'

'Look, Padma, Talking to the Baby in the Womb works magic! Nobody understands and responds to the wishes of a mother better than the child in her womb.'

'Is that so?'

'Yes. This is the most authentic information I can give you. Talk to your baby! Request your baby to stay safe, strong and intact, no matter how badly you vomit. Also, tell the baby to help you by controlling your nausea and vomiting.'

'Ma, this is the first time I am hearing something as new as this. It sounds weird. Will my baby understand if I talk to it? It's still a small foetus. I can't see it.'

'First of all, stop underestimating the life in you, dear. You are not carrying something that is devoid of emotions or lack of understanding! Babies in the womb are very sensitive, responsive, understanding and powerful life forms right from the stage of foetus!'

'Wow! It feels good already as I have been given a new dimension of thinking about the life growing in my womb, Ma!'

'Good! Now carry the good feeling forward and place your problems before your baby and request it to help you in easing your vomiting and stay strong!'

'How to talk to the baby, Ma?'

'Just talk to your baby the way you are talking to me now. Feel confident and respect the baby in your womb. As you try, you will see the result through your own experience. You will then not need any recommendations from me. Trust your baby, dear!'

'Sure, Ma.'

That night, Padma speaks to her baby in her womb.

'Sweetheart, this is the first time I am talking to you consciously. It feels

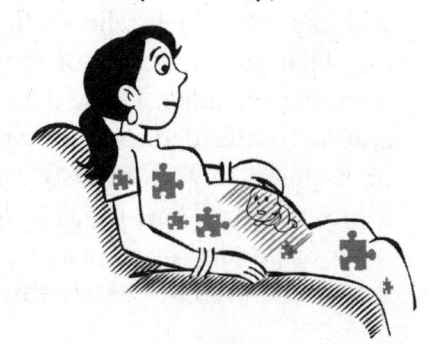

really good talking to you, though I am not sure if you understand me. Even before I start my darling, you mean so much to me! Right from the moment I conceived you, you have become my dream, my world. I love you so much that I am literally breathing you. Right now, I am worried about nausea. My condition hasn't improved in spite of medication. I'm feeling scared. You know, the doctor told me that if my vomiting doesn't subside, you might not stay with me. On hearing this, I felt very sad. My ma, your grandmother, advised me to talk to you. I have one request for you. Please stay strong, stay with me till the ninth month! No matter what, I want to deliver you safely into this world. Please stay put, hold on! And please help Mommy by reducing and controlling the vomiting through your love! I trust you completely, my darling! You may love me as much as I love you! Stay strong! I love you the most!'

After hearing Padma's story, a stunned Sheela asks, 'Oh my God! You literally spoke that to your foetus in your womb! Then what happened?'

'Yeah, Doctor and my ma gave me a precious gift in the form of advice that evening! After the heartfelt talk with my baby, I felt relieved that my baby is there with me. That gave me a lot of moral support. My fear of vomiting subsided. In the next two days, my vomiting gradually subsided. Not only that, while I was resting or napping, my mom also used to talk to my baby in my womb. That, too, yielded the best results! My baby responded and I was normal like anybody else. I delivered my baby safely through a normal delivery!

My husband was so grateful to my mom. Most of all, today my daughter is blooming into a strong athlete! Her immunity levels are very high.'

'Amazing!'

'So, are you not amazed at your own experiences with your baby?'

'Of course, I am but . . .'

'Self-doubt is an enemy to everyone, but to pregnant women it is the arch enemy! Please drive it out of your mind, when it is at its weakest, and it appears to be so now!'

'Oh, thank you very much, Padma! What an awesome favour you have bestowed on me! I see a ray of hope. I am grateful for your invaluable guidance!'

'Any time, Sheela! Now start talking to your baby and enjoy the sweetest results!'

'Sure, Padma! See you soon!'

A few days later, the buzzer rings at Sheela's house. Sheela opens the door and is pleasantly surprised to see Padma standing outside with healthy goodies in hand. Sheela welcomes her into her house. The two friends settle down comfortably for a hearty chat.

'How are you feeling now, Sheela?'

'I was about to tell you, Padma, my vomiting has almost stopped! Thanks for teaching the technique of Talking to the Baby in the Womb.

My baby is my saviour these days! I talked to my baby and my baby seems to take care of me from inside my womb! It's all awesomely magical, but still very practical! Talking to the Baby in the Womb works wonders! It's unbelievable, but true. Babies favour their moms like nobody else can ever do. What an amazing experience! I want every woman on earth to have this wonderful experience.'

'Yes, Sheela, so do I! I look forward to meeting you and your healthy baby, delivered normally, soon!'

'Thank you, Padma! My baby has heard you now, so my baby will make you smile as per your wish!'

NVP (Nausea and Vomiting during Pregnancy)

Morning Sickness

Pregnancy is a natural phenomenon and the body undergoes many miraculous changes internally. There are some special changes that are unique to pregnancy. Nausea and vomiting are two such important changes that are part of pregnancy. As such, there is nothing to worry about when it is mild to moderate nausea and vomiting. It doesn't harm the foetus in any way. It is quite normal for a pregnant woman to vomit and the frequency varies from woman to woman. For most women, vomiting might be there only up to three months, while for a few others, it may be there till the ninth month. Slight vomiting (about 50 per cent) is common and is considered as a symptom of pregnancy. It is, in fact, the natural reaction of the body due to certain hormonal changes that are special and specific to pregnancy.

Possible causes of vomiting include:

1. Human chorionic gonadotropin (hCG): This hormone rises rapidly during early pregnancy. Vomiting tends to peak around the same time as levels of hCG soar. What's more, conditions in which women have higher levels of hCG, such as twins or vesicular mole (GTN), usually have higher rates of nausea and vomiting.
2. A sensitive stomach: Some women's digestive tracts are more sensitive to the changes that happen during early pregnancy.
3. Stress: Some researchers have proposed that certain women are psychologically predisposed to having nausea and vomiting during pregnancy as an abnormal response to stress. However, there's no conclusive evidence to support this theory. Of course, if you're constantly nauseated or vomiting a lot, you certainly may begin to feel more stressed!
4. Allergic or immunological basis and neurogenic element also seem to play a role in NVP.

Severe Cases of Vomiting

For some women, vomiting during early pregnancy can be very severe. And those women need to take treatment to reduce severity, which otherwise will weaken the expecting mother. Hyperemesis gravidarum is the most severe form of vomiting that incapacitates the mother in her day-to-day activities, calls for hospitalization and vigorous treatment with intravenous fluids and other medications.

Treatment

Observations and Dietary Advice

Usually, frequent small meals (dry toast), crackers/biscuits, sips of water, plenty of rest and avoidance of fatty meals and spicy foods, along with reassurance is enough to relieve the symptom in a majority of mild cases. Avoid fried foods, strong odours, perfume, etc. Safe medicines in the form of injection, tablets

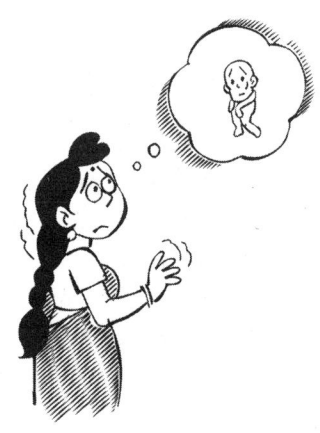

Baby small, weak and lean

and syrup are advised in mild to moderate cases. The pregnant woman is asked to keenly observe the food items that cause vomiting and avoid them. To ensure that her sugar level remains normal, she should frequently take small meals that don't induce vomiting. When the expectant mother skips her food for a long time due to fear of vomiting, the blood sugar levels fall and the resultant low sugar may cause severe and prolonged vomiting. Severe vomiting also exhausts her, and she will feel demoralized. Intravenous (IV) fluids and injections are given in such cases to control dehydration and vomiting. Many a time, I have found a strong emotional underlying cause in severe and persistent vomiting. Let us see some real-life examples.

Tanuja came to me in her sixth month of pregnancy with a history of persistent and severe vomiting since early pregnancy. She was very weak and frail as she was not taking sufficient food out of fear of vomiting. While I was examining her, I asked her whether she was keen about her pregnancy. Immediately her face brightened up and she said that she loved her husband so much and wanted this child to be a good gift for him. She was worried about the health of her baby, because of her continued vomiting. She added that she would do anything to have a healthy child. I asked her to take food and not worry or fear about vomiting.

Even if she vomited 90 per cent of her food, 10 per cent would go to her baby. If she increased the frequency of her food intake, that would be sufficient for the baby. Her baby would be healthy. She appeared relieved and said, 'Your words have removed my worry about my baby. It was an unbearable burden. Now I feel light.' After four days when Tanuja came back, she looked much better. Her vomiting had subsided substantially.

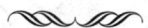

Rani came to me in the third month of her pregnancy. She complained of severe vomiting for the past two days and extreme pain in her abdomen. I immediately gave her IV fluids and injections, but there was no improvement. Her pain continued to be severe and it became unbearable—so much so that she started to roll on the floor. I asked her mother whether anything was bothering her, and she said that Rani was missing her husband very much. I asked her husband to come immediately. He came after a few hours. The next day, I was surprised to see a happy and cheerful Rani. She said she did not feel any pain and had regular food in the afternoon without vomiting. Her vomiting had totally subsided. She came only for her delivery. Sometimes, emotional disturbances too can lead to severe vomiting. Vomiting was due to the effect of 'pangs of separation' for Rani and the 'joy of reunion' stopped her vomiting dramatically.

What Are the Emotional Causes for the Persistence of Severe Vomiting?

Anxiety About the Health of the Baby

Generally, pregnant women feel anxious that vomiting may affect the health of the foetus. This makes them worry and the vomiting becomes persistent. If they are reassured that the baby would not be affected, they feel

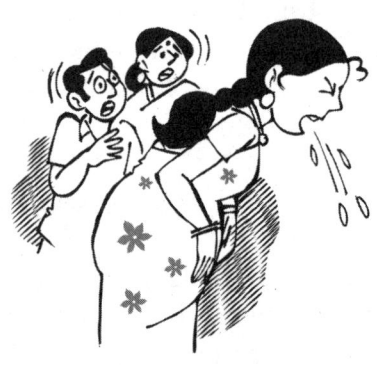

Anxiety of onlookers increases the chances of vomiting

relieved and eventually the vomiting stops. The power of love overcomes the fear of vomiting. In most cases, when she receives an authentic explanation that mild to moderate vomiting is not harmful, she accepts vomiting as part of her pregnancy and is able to overcome the fear of vomiting. Vomiting can be controlled through understanding, positive attitude, diet changes and medicines.

Embarrassment and Fear of Vomiting

Embarrassment caused by vomiting in front of others is common in civilized society. It is the habit to conform to social etiquette. When a pregnant woman develops fear that she would vomit every time she takes some food, and stops taking food; vomiting becomes persistent. They need to overcome inhibitions and feel emotionally free and not feel guilty about vomiting in front of others.

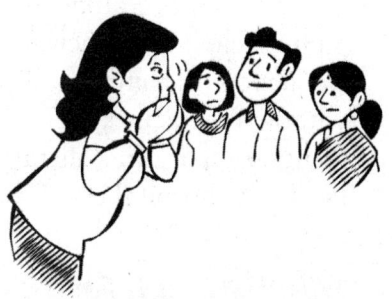

Feeling guilty for vomiting in front of others

During pregnancy, mothers need to be re-educated through awareness and counselling. Vomiting is part of pregnancy, and it will slowly subside if we don't pay much attention; it will not harm us. If we worry about it, it persists. It's like the thorn in the rose plant.

How Did Our Elders Manage Vomiting Effectively?

Our elders calmed expectant mothers down by saying things like 'Marriage and vomiting can't be stopped'. So, what cannot be cured must be endured; that positive state of acceptance of vomiting reduced the anxiety, guilt, fear and hence frequency of vomiting. They could manage vomiting without medicines very effectively just by proper mental preparation, dietary advice and moral support in the pre-hospital era.

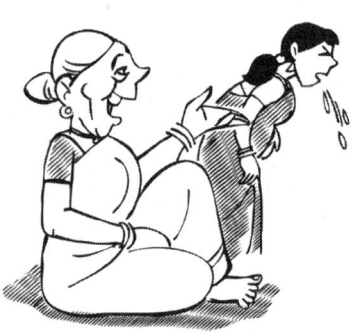

Reassuring grandmother

What Happens If Fear Is Not Removed?

If they continue to live in fear, their vomiting will persist and become more severe. They will feel completely out of control, leading to anticipation of a negative outcome. And expectedly, in most cases, complications creep in and pregnancy becomes a great burden. Sometimes this may lead to miscarriage.

Doctor: According to Rudyard Kipling, 'Words are, of course, the most powerful drug used by mankind.'

Hope it was informative and useful. I'm sure you will agree with Rudyard Kipling.

Sahana: Thanks, Aunty. Now I understand vomiting is not a big issue; it is a natural occurrence during pregnancy. It is not going to bother me if I stop worrying and make suitable dietary adjustments and take medicines. With Talking to the Baby in the Womb in my pregnancy toolkit, I can handle it comfortably.

Vijaya: Andal, now I understand the secret of my mother's relaxed attitude about vomiting. I like your approach of combining modern technology with the wisdom of the ancient times. From now on I, too, will join her in supporting Sahana. My mother would be interested in discussing these experiences with you.

Doctor: 'Vijaya, please don't hesitate to bring your mother next time. It has been a long time since I met her. It'll be great, talking to her about these things and knowing about her experiences. Sahana, we'll talk about nutrition next time. Bye!

Sahana: Okay, Aunty.

Sometimes the strength of motherhood is greater than natural laws.

I KNOW HOW MUCH HE LOVES ME WHEN HE HOLDS THE BOWL WHEN I'M VOMITING

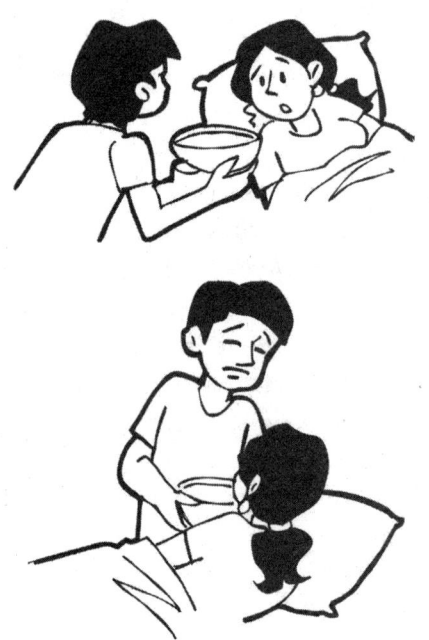

EVEN THOUGH HE CAN'T STAND THE SIGHT OF VOMIT

9

Meditation and Yoga

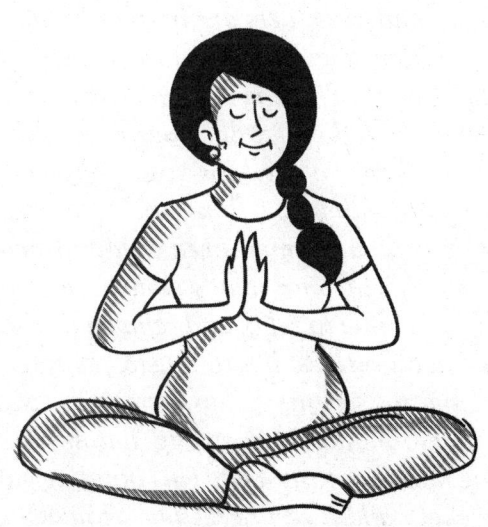

Sahana: Hello, Aunty! I'm meeting you after a gap of four months. I'm fine, aunty. As suggested by you, I have been practising the Talk to the Baby in the Womb technique and the baby is responding well, and I'm feeling well connected with the baby. Pregnancy feels like an easy and enjoyable journey with the baby. I'm so happy and confident after practising the Talking to the Baby in the Womb technique. All my tests are normal.

Doctor: That's good. I'm glad about your awareness, Sahana.

Sahana: Aunty, I have a doubt about my friend Bhavana, who is in the fourth month of pregnancy. She lives in Delhi and her elders are in their hometown far away. She is jittery these days and I counsel her on and off over the phone. There is a yoga centre nearby. She wants to know whether it will be useful for her. Aunty, do you think there is a need for yoga and meditation?

Doctor: Yes, Sahana, I think these days everyone, particularly pregnant women, need yoga and meditation. In the olden days, life moved at a slow pace. People had plenty of leisure time to relax and rejuvenate themselves by taking a lively interest in art, music, reading, reciting and listening to scriptures, prayers, etc. Moreover, interpersonal bonding was strong within the family and among neighbours as well. This bonding gave them mental strength and a secure feeling. Nowadays, life is moving at a fast pace; there is really no time to stand and stare. Family ties have become weak. We are too happy to have hundreds of friends on Facebook but we pay little attention to building bosom friendship. Since everyone in the race needs to have some way of recharging their energy, yoga and meditation seem to fit the bill. They are particularly useful and necessary in pregnancy, because pregnancy comes with a bundle of emotions. One may feel happy, sad, excited and worried all in the span of a few minutes. This is due to the pregnancy hormones, along with the changes in lifestyle, sleep disturbances and the responsibility of welcoming a new member into the family. It can leave one feeling anxious and even stressed in the midst of all the positives because of the changes in the thinking pattern in the family and society.

In the old days, elders in the joint family, who had attended several deliveries, by virtue of their keen observation, clearly understood the impact of emotions on pregnancy. The enormous emotional support of the elders at home, offered with conviction and confidence in the form of proverbs and stories, allayed the anxiety and tension about pregnancy and delivery. Physical activity in the form of household work was insisted upon. Elders played the role of a seasoned counsellor and an efficient nurse. Thus, low-risk pregnant mothers had an easy, normal delivery with little medical help because of proper physical and mental preparation.

With modernization, lifestyle has changed; a majority of women are working and have to balance their career and family. Besides, the number of joint families is fast dwindling, yielding place to nuclear families. There is no one at home to give physical and emotional support. Hence, pregnancy is perceived as an additional burden. The vast and rapid cultural changes in society are greatly influencing modern mothers. A career woman can be most efficient in her physical and mental capabilities. This speed has made her emotionally vulnerable and sensitive. In the name of diplomacy and decorum, there is a constant effort at suppressing emotional upsurges.

She feels too shy and inhibited to express her doubt, fear, anxiety or worry to others for fear of being misunderstood. Such demanding situations throw her emotionally off balance, and she does not have sufficient time to heal herself efficiently. These pent-up emotions are the most important factors for causing stress-related health problems in pregnancy, such as pregnancy-induced hypertension, diabetes and intrauterine growth restriction. Most of the knowledge about delivery is acquired from hearsay, interaction with relatives and friends, newspapers, TV, the cinema and social media. They depict all deliveries as difficult with unbearable pain. This is only information—not fact—because some deliveries are difficult and some are easy; the reason why it is difficult and when it is easy, is not explored at all. Due to small family size and increase in the incidence of infertility, every child has become precious. Hence the expecting mother is more concerned about her own health and that of the baby, along with a fear and doubt about her capabilities of coping with delivery pain and not expressing it.

Sahana: Very true, Aunty. It's like you are reading their mind. Doctor: Yes. That's how I learnt about the language of emotions.

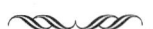

Even though there have been great advances in technology, all deliveries are not as smooth as they should be. This is mainly due to an increase in the mother's stress and anxiety, while the physical aspects of pregnancy, in the form of tests and treatment, are very well taken care of, the emotional well-being of the expecting mother is totally neglected, making pregnancy more stressful; the irony is that in the pre-hospital era, pregnancy was sheer joy and women could have as many children as they wanted. The extinction of the species of supportive and resourceful elders has created a vacuum that needs to be filled. As there is no medicine to create happiness or decrease anxiety and worry, there is an urgent need for an effective self-help tool to address the stress. Our age-old Indian tradition of meditation and yoga is a powerful tool that can to a great extent fill the gap, enabling the mother to restore peace and tranquillity.

Let Us See What Meditation Is

It involves focusing attention, for a set period of time, on breath, a mantra (repeated positive phrase) or the present moment. It helps in finding inner peace, and getting in touch with the inner self through mental focus.

There are different types of meditation:

- Mindfulness meditation is a form of meditation where you focus on the physical and emotional sensations that are going on in the present moment without judging how they make you feel.

- Transcendental Meditation involves repeating a mantra silently.
- Heartfulness meditation is focusing on the heart.
- They have a special programme for expectant mothers. The Heartfulness Institute in association with IAP has formed Mission Lakshya 1000. It believes in providing nutrition with a nurturing environment in the critical period of the first 1000 days starting from preconception through pregnancy up to two years of life. They associate themselves with the pregnant mother in her journey, helping her maximize the child's potential; thereby, the nation's future.
- Walking meditation is a kind of meditation where you walk mindfully for a fixed amount of time. You may choose to focus on your breath or your steps.
- Deep breathing is one of the most effective ways to ease muscle tension, lower heart rate and help fall asleep. It requires the expecting mother to breathe deeply and rhythmically. Breathe slowly through the nose for four seconds, keeping the mouth closed. Be conscious of your stomach rising as you gradually fill the lungs and diaphragm with air, then hold for one second before exhaling through the nose to the count of four. It can be done at any time and in any posture.
- Body scanning is a form of progressive relaxation that involves sitting or lying down while focusing on various parts of the body and breathing into those places of tension that need to be released.
- Progressive muscle relaxation is a technique that includes body-scanning meditation, and may take

a couple of weeks to master. It's like a natural sleeping pill, which one really appreciates as the pregnancy progresses and a good night's sleep becomes more and more elusive. Here's how to do it: lie down on the bed or on the floor and tense the muscles completely, then let them totally relax. Focus on one muscle group at a time and alternate between the left and right sides of your body. One possible route is to start by tensing and releasing the hand and forearm muscles, followed by the triceps and biceps, then the face, the chest and shoulders, stomach, legs, and finally, the feet.

- Guided imagery or visualization is another way of effective meditation. Just picture yourself in a place you find peaceful or relaxing: a tropical beach, a flower-filled meadow or wherever your own private bliss may be. Next, imagine every detail of that place, from the sounds to the smells and everything in between. An alternative to this technique is to think of an image from a magazine or photograph and fill in every detail in your mind. Visualization takes some practice, but once you get it, you'll find it's a great way to quieten your mind, ease your tension and help you drift off to sleep.

When done consistently over an extended period of time, meditation can have a host of positive benefits, physical and mental, for the expectant moms. There are many benefits, both physical and mental to both mother and the baby. Scientific studies have proven the efficacy of yoga and meditation in pregnancy.

1) Meditation can help with pregnancy symptoms, including fatigue, mood changes and sleep disturbances.
2) Studies have found that meditation and other mindfulness-based exercises during pregnancy reduce anxiety, depression and perceived stress.
3) It helps in reducing post-delivery depression.
4) It removes fear and pain associated with childbirth. It reduces perceptions of the pain and length of labour.
5) Body awareness can also be vital in helping pregnant women notice early on if something doesn't feel quite right, like leaking of amniotic fluid and decrease in foetal movement. This helps in taking treatment early, which may be a very crucial step in preventing serious complications for the mother and the baby.
6) Yoga and meditation significantly improve birth weight, prevent premature births, and reduce medical complications for the mother and the baby.

Let us see the results of studies done about the efficacy of meditation in pregnancy.

Mood Changes: Anxiety and Depression

Anxiety means tension, restlessness, difficulty in concentrating, and fear that something bad is going to happen, etc. Depression is reflected in a depressed mood, lack of interest in enjoyable activities, decrease in appetite and sleep. Feeling guilty or worthless, etc. Meditation can help us feel refreshed, rejuvenated and a bit more focused, ready to tackle that never-ending to-do list. Studies show that after meditation, participants developed positive feelings such as enjoyment, gratitude, and hope.

They also observed positive changes in their behaviour in day-to-day life. Participants talked about learning to stop struggling and accepting things as they are; They remembered to stop and breathe, and then take conscious action rather than acting out of anger or frustration.

A 2012 study of an eight-week mindfulness programme found reduction in depression, stress and anxiety compared with a control group.

Studies on 1) the levels of hormones and 2) specific brain areas have revealed interesting findings that lead to changes in the mental state and behaviour due to meditation.[*]

Effect on Hormones

Sleep

Melatonin is a naturally occurring hormone that is key to induce sleep. Rutgers University researchers found that meditation boosted melatonin levels. It's a common observation; many people slip into sleep while meditating.

---

[*] Newman, Kira M. 'Four Reasons to Practice Mindfulness during Pregnancy' Greater Good Magazine 17 August 2016, https://greatergood.berkeley.edu/article/item/four_reasons_to_practice_mindfulness_during_pregnancy, accessed on 11 July 2025.

A highly-referenced University of California-Davis study showed a drop in cortisol levels by staggering amounts of 50 per cent plus! Meditation supercharges the mom's body with neuro-transmitter serotonin, a happy hormone.[*]

Pain during Childbirth

In 2001, a randomized, double-blind study of seventy-eight volunteers, researchers from Wake Forest University (Zeiden et al) found that after only four days of meditation training, the subjects could handle pain 27 per cent better than the control group.[†]

Meditation Boosts Two Natural Painkillers: Endorphins and Dopamine

Endorphins, which are upto one hundred times more powerful than the strongest painkiller, morphine, are released in abundance both during and after meditation. Dopamine, a chemical messenger known for numbing pain, is another chemical very helpful in the delivery room.

---

[*] Jacobs, T.L., Shaver, P.R., Epel, E.S., et al. 'Self-reported mindfulness and cortisol during a Shamatha meditation retreat', *Health Psychology*, Vol. 32, no. 10 (2013), pp. 1104-9.

[†] F. Zeidan, et al. 'Mindfulness Meditation-Based Pain Relief Employs Different Neural Mechanisms Than Placebo and Sham Mindfulness Meditation-Induced Analgesia', *Journal of Neuroscience*, Vol. 35, no. 46 (2015), 10.1523/JNEUROSCI.2542-15.2015, accessed on 11 July 2025.

Effect on Brain Centres

Research has found that meditation activates the brain's 'happy centre', the prefrontal cortex. Meditation strengthens and literally 'grows' the brain region, which shrinks when we get depressed, the hippocampus. Meditation quietens the brain's 'fight or flight' stress centre, the amygdala.[*]

Effect on Baby

A study found that for 169 pregnant women, a daily yoga and meditation practice significantly improved birth weight, reduced premature births and lessened the overall medical complications for the newborn.[†]

In a 2005 study of 335 pregnant women in Bengaluru, India, half of them were assigned to practise yoga and meditation while the other half walked for an hour per day, starting in their second trimester and continuing until delivery. The yoga group, who attended yoga classes for a week and then practised at home, had fewer premature births and fewer babies with low birthweight.[‡]

---

[*] Goleman, Daniel, and Davidson, Richard J. *Altered Traits: Science Reveals How Meditation Changes Your Mind, Brain, and Body* (New York: Avery, 2017); Davidson, R.J., Kabat-Zinn, J., et al. 'Alterations in brain and immune function produced by mindfulness meditation', *Psychosomatic Medicine*, Vol. 65, no. 4 (July–August 2003).

[†] Narendran, S., Nagarathna, R., et al. 'Efficacy of yoga on pregnancy outcome', *Journal of Alternative Complementary Medicine*, Vol. 11, no. 2 (April 2005), pp. 237–44.

[‡] Newman, 'Four Reasons', 2016.

In 2011, a northern Thailand study showed only 6 per cent of women in a meditation group delivered their babies prematurely, compared with the 16 per cent in the care-as-usual group.*

In a 2015 study from the Netherlands, babies whose mothers did meditation during pregnancy, at ten months, were less likely to have difficulties settling down and adjusting to new environments ('self-regulation') or controlling their attention and behaviour ('effortful control'). For example, the babies might be more likely to calm down faster after crying or keep their hands off things they are not supposed to touch.†

Doctor: Now we understand the effectiveness of meditation in uplifting emotional well-being of mother, ensuring smooth and pleasant journey of pregnancy and delivery.

Sahana: Thanks a lot, Aunty, for the valuable information about meditation. Can you please enlighten me on yoga?

Doctor: Sahana, do you know the birthplace of yoga is our motherland

Bharath, i.e. India? Patanjali Maharishi introduced this system many centuries ago. But it's the West that took a keen interest in it, evaluated through studies, the efficacy and usefulness of yoga in health and propagated it. We should be proud that the Swami Vivekananda Yoga

---

* Ibid.
† Ibid.

Anusandhana Samasthana, an esteemed yoga research centre in Bengaluru, India, is doing commendable work on yoga and alternative systems of medicine.
We will now see the benefits of yoga in pregnancy.

Yoga helps reduce stress, both physical and mental. It creates internal awareness that enables one to recognize, clearly, inner conflict and stress and develop inner stamina to face one's problems. It also makes the body relaxed. It gives deep rest and relaxation to every cell in the body, thereby setting right the disturbed internal function. It rejuvenates the tired organs through promoting the parasympathetic tone.

Benefits of Yoga

Yoga helps improve sleep, relieves back pain, improves flexibility, strength and endurance—all these together make for easy delivery, lower risk of IUGR by increasing placental circulation. These also lower the risk of gestational hypertension and diabetes in the mother. Though there are many yoga exercises that can be done during pregnancy, I would like to suggest three important pelvic yoga asanas.

Butterfly Exercise: Baddha Konasana

Technique: Slowly bend the knees and bring the soles of your feet together at a comfortable distance from your body. Later, after you have relaxed a little, you can draw them closer. Hold your feet with both hands. Gently bounce your knees up and down, using the elbows as levers to press the feet.

Do not use any force. Repeat up to twenty to thirty times. Straighten your legs and relax. If your thighs are not touching or are close to the floor, then you can place a soft cushion underneath each knee for support.

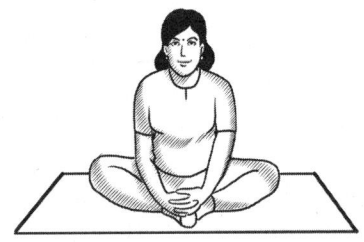

Sitting perpendicular to the ground

Benefits: It increases suppleness of the joints, widening the pelvic diameters. Poses are excellent for loosening up the hip joint, and help a woman get used to the feeling of opening up. Can increase blood circulation to the pelvic floor. It relaxes the pelvic floor muscles. They also help relieve tension and tiredness from inner thigh muscles and legs.

Squatting: Malasana

It is also the garland pose.

Technique:

- You need to stand with your feet wider than your hips and inhale

- As you exhale, you must bend your knees as low as you can so that your buttocks are only two or three inches above the ground.
- Bring your hands together in a prayer position and lean forward to balance.
- Hold for a couple of minutes and let it relax.

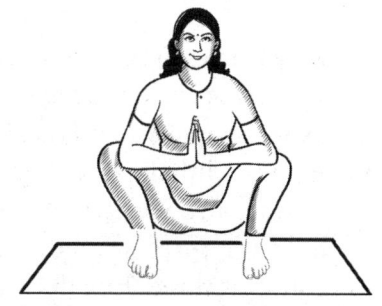

Benefits: Squatting regularly helps increase the mobility of your pelvic and hip joints. When we squat, muscles in the back, buttocks and pelvic floor lengthen and relax, while the muscles in front of the body contract.

In this position, the pelvic floor relaxes and the blood supply to the whole pelvic area improves. The perineal tissues relax and can stretch evenly when we squat, so regular practice may help to prevent tearing in the final stages of the birth.

The full squat pose strengthens legs, thighs, calves, feet and ankles.

AP diameter of pelvic outlet widens and as much as 30 per cent of the sacrum is free to move.

The squatting position is effective in shortening the second stage of labour, which is why it is jokingly called the midwives' forceps.

Kegel Exercise:

Technique:

- Kegel exercises are easy to do. It's all about squeezing and relaxing the same muscles you would use to stop a stream of urine and motion.
- As you inhale, draw your pelvic floor muscles upwards towards your uterus, contract them and hold for three seconds at a time, then relax for a count of three. Exhale and relax.
- Repeat this three times a day. Aim for at least three sets of ten to fifteen repetitions a day. At first, you may find it easier to practise lying down. Later on, you'll be able to do them lying down, standing or even while sitting.

Benefits:

- Problems caused by weakness of the pelvic floor, such as prolapse of the uterus, bowel or bladder can be prevented or reduced by this exercise.
- Varicosities can be relieved.
- The exercise also improves blood circulation to this area and reduces the risk of perineum tearing or injury during the birth.
- Knowing how to relax your pelvic floor muscles is very helpful when your baby is being born and the head needs to pass through these muscles (internal rotation). Practised daily during pregnancy, the pelvic floor exercise greatly reduces the risk

of damage to the pelvic floor during birth and promotes rapid recovery postnatally.
- Resume daily practice as soon as possible after the birth and continue for a few weeks thereafter. The pelvic floor exercise should be practised regularly throughout a woman's life.

Though there are many yoga asanas that can be practised from the early stages of pregnancy, I would advise only three asanas for childbirth, to be done from the end of the eighth month or the beginning of the ninth. I find that one or two weeks of pelvic exercise facilitates normal delivery. I must tell you that there is a group of sceptical people, who anticipate negative outcomes like premature delivery and miscarriage and attribute it to exercises.

So, it is always better to take doctor's advice about exercises.

Sahana: Do you think yoga, like antenatal checkup, is a must for all pregnant mothers?

Doctor: Yoga is very useful for the expecting mother. I want you to remember, every pregnant mother is the best mother and every child is the best for the mother, whether endorsed by others or not. Also, every pregnancy experience can be different for the same mother. Every mother has her own preferences and beliefs. Once she understands this, she accepts herself and stress is less. When we insist on something, and if the mother is not able to do it, she feels guilty and that is more harmful. The best results are seen when they take whatever diet or whatever exercise they are able to do willingly and happily. That's why I don't insist on anything. I give suggestions and strongly recommend yoga and meditation and leave it to their choice. In this context, let me tell you the well-known story of Vinayaka and Subrahmanya Swami.

Sahana: Please explain, Aunty.

Doctor: To get a mango, Vinayaka, who strongly believed that his parents were his universe, immediately went around them. Subrahmanya literally went around the world. Both ways are effective. One is mental and the other is physical. It's the belief and faith in the path that makes success possible. I have seen it myself many a time. It's the confidence rather than the method that matters. Some feel household work is very effective and enough; some swear that only walking or yoga helped them deliver easily. I give them the freedom to choose their option and stick to it. Here it would be pertinent to quote Hippocrates, the fourth century BC Greek physician who is regarded as the father of medicine, 'It is more important to know what sort of a person has the disease than to know what sort of disease the person has.

Sahana: For a normal delivery, which exercise holds the magic key?

Doctor: Let's first know why they want a normal delivery and what it means to them and later how.

Some want normal delivery because

1) It's a natural process

2) Some want it to avoid Caesarean section, as they believe that after a surgery, health suffers a setback
3) Others want normal delivery for want of family help at home or because they have to go back to their job after delivery.

They believe that if they have a normal delivery, they can look after themselves and the baby well, without anyone else's assistance. In family circles, normal delivery is perceived as a success and Caesarean section as a failure. It is also a short-term goal, as nobody will ask about the mode of delivery after one month. I have seen some mothers feel bad and guilty, in spite of having a healthy baby, as the elders in the family are unhappy about Caesarean section. We need to understand that people are different from their beliefs. We should certainly respect elders for their relationship and age, but need not respect all their beliefs. Differing from their belief does not amount to disrespecting them. If we understand this, we will not feel guilty about differing from their belief system. The stress of making them happy and being in their good books by having a normal delivery will not be there anymore. This lack of anxiety can result in normal delivery, while stress and anxiety of satisfying them by having a normal delivery is more likely to result in caesarean section.

Setback in the health of the mother or the baby is the real failure, because it can have long term impact. It can result in strained relationship among family members. Caesarean section at the right time will not only save a life but retain good health of baby in many instances. The benefit of caesarean section outweighs the risk when it comes to safety of baby or mother. Therefore, our primary goal must be a healthy and happy mother and baby, and C-section is really helpful to achieve that goal whenever the situation demands it. Mode of delivery is a secondary goal.

Sahana: A very valuable point for me, Aunty. Thanks a lot.

Doctor: We also must know when and why Caesarean section is done.

Elective Caesarean section is done before the onset of delivery pains.

Indications:

- CPD baby malpresentation: breech, transverse lie, big baby, cephalo pelvic disproportion or IUGR (Intrauterine growth restriction)
- Placenta previa—type III and IV. Placenta in the lower segment instead of the upper
- Maternal disease: GDM (gestational diabetes mellitus), high blood sugar, PET (pre-eclamptic toxaemia), high BP, as advised by the condition of patient.

Emergency Caesarean section—trial for normal delivery is allowed and when it becomes necessary for the mother or the baby, Caesarean section is resorted to.

1) Caesarean section is done when health of the baby is at risk—heartbeat variation, baby passing motion (meconium) before birth.

2) Mother: There is no progress–cervix is not opening up or cervical dystocia
3) Baby's head not descending due to the position of the head, presenting diameter of foetal head, big baby, etc.

For any safe, normal delivery, the requirements are

1) Average baby weight
2) Dilatation of the cervix
3) Descent of the head
4) Baby's well-being

For normal delivery, the limiting step is dilatation of the cervix (opening of uterus). The opening of the cervix depends on the mental state of the mother. If the mother is happy, relaxed, confident and secure, the cervix becomes soft and short and opens easily without causing much pain and shortens duration of delivery. Sometimes she is scared, anxious or apprehensive about labour pains because of the impact of movies and magazines or horror birth stories, or she may also have a doubt or a strong negative belief that she can't have a normal delivery. In these conditions, the cervix becomes rigid, long and thick, causing more pain and requiring more pressure. Hence the mother has to undergo prolonged and difficult labour.

The take-home message is when the baby is of average weight, whether the delivery is easy or difficult is directly dependent on the mindset of the mother, indirectly on family and society, who influence her beliefs. Expecting mothers should be frank in expressing their doubts or fears to the family or the medical team and getting them cleared to become relaxed and have an easy normal delivery.

Let's see some of the common negative beliefs.

(a) Her friends and cousins or mother had Caesarean section.
(b) Doubt that she is not young enough to have a normal delivery.
(c) The family's perception that she is too thin or weak to withstand pain.

Sahana: Interesting, Aunty. So, what is the secret code for safe and easy normal delivery?

Doctor: It involves physical and mental preparation. We will now see physical preparation.

We advise the mothers to do walking, breathing and household work from the beginning. The best ninth-month pelvic exercises are butterfly, squatting and kegel exercises.

During delivery, leave all your problems to the doctor and the team. If necessary, accept Caesarean section willingly for the sake of a healthy baby. This is an important tip for the mother to overcome anxiety and be relaxed during delivery. Also, if there is no progress and she ends up in Caesarean section, the mother should not feel bad as though she has failed; she should have the satisfaction that she tried her best to have a normal delivery and gave her best to the baby. Regular exercise and yoga are good and helpful.

But positive belief is even more powerful. I know of women who were scared even to take an injection, have had easy, normal delivery.

This was because they had strong faith and felt secure with their husband, family members and the medical team, baby or god. In some cases, they had not done any physical exercise, nor any household work. I reckoned that this was so because of the power of positive feelings in them. In sharp contrast.

If the mother has a negative mindset (fear, anxiety or negative beliefs), delivery is more painful, difficult and prolonged.

Absolute faith / trust / belief: Some mothers have immense confidence in themselves or strong trust in others. They strongly believe that normal delivery is very much possible and don't even entertain the slightest doubt about the probability of Caesarean Section. Mostly they will have normal delivery. Healing and recovery will also be good.

When the belief is not so strong. I come across two types of situations.

It depends on acceptance of Caesarean section:

a) Belief not strong along with acceptance of Caesarean section

Mother wants normal delivery and is

- Willing to try for it.
- Not confident about having normal delivery.

- Wholeheartedly willing for Caesarean section if the situation demands.
- She is not anxious, but calm and relaxed—cervix is favourable.
- Many times, normal delivery occurs.
- Sometimes emergency Caesarean section becomes mandatory.
- Even after surgery the mother is happy.
- Healing and recovery are good.

The proverb 'Hope for the best and be prepared for the worst' clearly explains this situation.

B) Belief not strong with non-acceptance of Caesarean Section.

- Mother wants only normal delivery.
- Not at all willing for Caesarean section.
- She is neither confident, nor has trust in the doctor.
- She is always gripped by anxiety and worry about the possibility of Caesarean section—cervix is unfavourable.
- She is most likely to land up having a Caesarean section.
- After surgery, she feels remorse and is unhappy.

In some cases, even though they had done yoga or exercises diligently, they could not have a normal delivery because of their negative beliefs and had no option except having a Caesarean section because of lack of progress or foetal distress.

Now let us see how strong belief helps in having a normal delivery and what happens when there is lack of strong belief. We will recollect about Belief from chapter one.

Belief is the feeling of certainty that it will happen. Belief is necessary to translate thinking into action, i.e. desired result.

We know that the rate-limiting step for the duration of labour is effacement (shortening) and opening up of the cervix—the mouth of the uterus. This effacement and dilatation of cervix is directly dependent on the mental state of the mother. so, if the mother is positive (happy, relaxed, confident, stress-free), delivery is easy, less painful and short.

There is another condition called wanting a Caesarean section. This needs to be differentiated from accepting Caesarean section.

Wanting Caesarean section means, mother wants only Caesarean section; she doesn't even think about normal delivery.

Wanting Caesarean Section = Wants only Caesarean Section. Willing and happy about it.

Acceptance of Caesarean Section = Wants Normal Delivery. Willing for Caesarean Section.

Non-Acceptance of Caesarean Section = Wants only Normal Delivery.
Not Willing for Caesarean Section.

So, the Final Formula

Physical: Diet, exercise, yoga and meditation, average weight of the baby and mother's pelvic adequate.

Mental: Have a mentor, do Talking to the Baby in the Womb, express and get doubts cleared in pregnancy and during delivery. Have a trustful birth companion, faith in the doctor and accept caesarean section wholeheartedly when it becomes necessary.

Sahana: I understood it's possible to have safe and easy normal delivery. I will be well prepared for normal delivery. It's okay if I land up in Caesarean section, as long as the baby and myself are healthy. Bonding with the baby and moulding the baby is more important than the mode of delivery.

Doctor: Perfect, Sahana, labour pains, breastfeeding and womb song are the gifts given to the baby only by the mother. Have a wonderful pregnancy and enjoy delivery, dear. God bless you!

Sahana: Thanks a lot, Aunty, for teaching and educating the expectant mothers and the family.

Doctor: Yes, Sahana, I feel truly indebted to the mothers from whose experience I have learnt these valuable lessons. That's why I am passionate about giving back to society. With these like-minded mothers, let us produce children infused with the spirit of Vivekananda's mother, Teresa and A.P.J.Abdul Kalam.

Sahana: Ah! Now I understand the secret of your passion. I'll join hands with you, Aunty, to continue the chain.

10

Nutrition and Diet

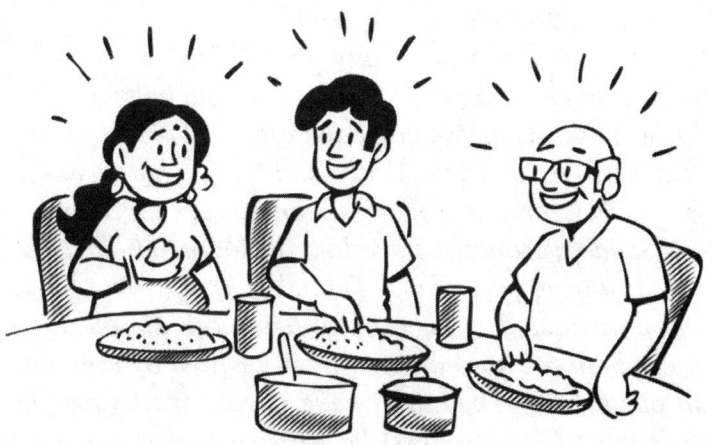

Eating is a need; enjoying the food is an art.

Sahana: Hello, Aunty, my grandma has come with me.

Doctor: Namaste, Lakshmi aunty. It has been ages since I saw you, your kammarkat *taste is the same. I enjoyed it.*

Lakshmi Aunty: I was also eager to see you, dear. After listening to your Talking to the Baby in the Womb technique, I wished, had I known it earlier, I could have practised it better. None the less, we too practised it. You know how? Our elders used to bless us, 'Dheergasumangali bhava! Suputrapropthirastu'. I used to believe it and remember it often, and that gave me a lot of secure feeling. That was an indirect way of Talking to the Baby in the Womb.

Doctor: Very true, Aunty, that's the reason why in spite of poverty, the world was a safer and happier place those days. Elders practised and preached moral values, and it was followed implicitly; and that's what I want to bring back through Talking to the Baby in the Womb.

Sahana: Aunty, I have lots of doubts about what to eat during pregnancy. Though I know some foods are nutritious, I am averse to them now, should I eat more than my normal quantity as insisted by everyone in our family? They say I have to eat for two people. Is it true? Please suggest healthy foods that I can eat during pregnancy.

Doctor: Yes, Sahana, we'll talk about feelings associated with food, foods that are mood stressors and supporters, and tips on what to eat and how to eat.

Sahana: What about the baby, Aunty?

Doctor: It is now widely accepted, Sahana, that what you eat affects your baby too, it may even be able to comprehend taste. Let's see the Story of Sanyukta.

Meera and Nivi are friends and are going out with Meera's daughter, Samyukta.

'Meera, why are we entering a health-food hub now?'

'It is because only here we shall be served sprouts and carrot juice, all fresh and made to order, Nivi.'

'But why on earth do we have to order sprouts and carrot juice? Have you forgotten that we have our little Samyukta with us?'

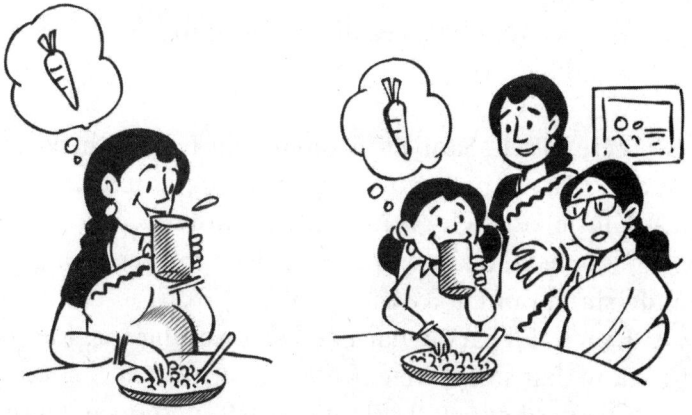

Both mother and daughter relishing carrot juice.

'How can any mother forget about her daughter? In fact, it is for Samyukta's sake that I am entering this food hub.'

'What are you saying? I don't understand!'

'Come along, yeah, this is the best spot for us three with one highchair. Let's sit here, Samyukta sweetheart. Here you go, see now you are seated in a highchair. Sit comfortably, dear. Take a look at the menu card and tick your orders. What am I to order, hmmm . . .'

'Here comes the waitress. Please order for me too. I am new to this place and I can't decide on the menu.'

'Good afternoon, Ma'am! May I take your orders, please?'

'A very good afternoon to you, Devi. Usual for me and Samyukta, for my friend here, who is new to this place, please bring one plate of veggie fruit green salad, one spinach smoothie and also bring two date delights.'

'You seem to be a regular at this hub.'

'Yes, Nivi, we are!'

'We?'

'Yes, myself, Samyukta and my husband, whenever he can spare time.' 'You bring Samyukta here? She is just a little kid! Why bring her here now?'

'You need to know the story from the beginning to understand our choice of this place.'

'Exactly! That's what I've been waiting for. I need to know that story, Meera.'

'Okay, okay, chill. Here comes our service, enjoy and listen to the story.'

'Here are your health menus, ladies, please enjoy!'

'Sure, Devi, thank you!'

'This is the first time that I am tasting this salad and fruit mix, and it is so delicious!'

'Our family favourite. It is a combo of fresh vegetables, greens and fruit mix with lemon and watermelon juices.'

'Yummy!'

'You enjoy and at the same time take a look at what my daughter is doing.' 'Samyukta dear, what are you eating now?'

'Sprouts and carrot juice.' 'Is this menu your favourite?'

'Yes, yummy in the tummy!'

'Ha! Now I get it. It's surprising! Your daughter is an angel, Meera! How can a child of this age enjoy sprouts and carrot juice so much? My twelve-year-old son runs away from broccoli and sprouts when I try to feed him! Since childhood, he has always enjoyed chips and fries!'

'Did you enjoy chips and fries when you were pregnant with your son?'

'Oh, yes, I used to eat plates and plates of chips when I was pregnant. Why do you ask me that now?'

'It's because of your love for chips and fries that your son has developed a strong liking for them. I still remember that you used to run away from healthy, natural food when you were pregnant and even before that, then why blame him?'

'Come on, Meera, what has my eating during pregnancy got to do with my son's preferences?'

'It has everything to do with what you eat during pregnancy.'

'Enlighten me on this, Meera.'

'Yes, Nivi. I will narrate my experience to you. You will be able to understand the connection automatically.

During my schooldays, I was an athlete and I used to have this liking for healthy food. I used to like sprouts and carrot juice and take them whenever I could. When I was pregnant, my husband too, was particular that I eat more healthy food that would nourish. My baby, too, informed me through her movements that she enjoyed sprouts and carrot juice very much!'

'Oh, did she?'

'Yes, of course. My husband and I started conscious parenting from the day my pregnancy was confirmed. Doctor Andal taught us "soul seeding" through the Talking to the Baby in the Womb technique. My husband and I took turns and talked to Samyukta while she was still in my womb. Both of us developed familiarity with Samyukta, which blossomed into understanding and companionship we cherished. Thus, the bonding got strengthened. It was only through her movements that I was able to know her tastes, likes and dislikes; she understood me and my husband perfectly well and we understood her fully; and even now she gets along with us very well. She can understand our feelings without verbal expression and respond very quickly and aptly.

After Samyukta started eating, she used to look at carrot juice with a certain fondness whenever I made it. I tried giving her a spoonful of carrot juice and she started asking for more. One day, I was eating sprouts for breakfast and Samyukta came near my plate and happily started eating the sprouts. At first, I was surprised. Then I consulted my doctor, and she told me that my eating habits had had a strong influence on Samyukta and it is quite natural and normal. From then on, my husband started hunting for a spot where we could go during the weekends, where we could relax, enjoy and eat healthy food and we came across this health-food hub. Now, you can see Samyukta finish her plate of sprouts and a full small glass of carrot juice without any fuss or help or persuasion from me. Now you got the story?'

'I feel bowled over! I am sorry now that I didn't pay heed to you or Mom when you encouraged me to eat a healthy, natural diet during my pregnancy.'

'It happens, Nivi, don't worry. It is okay to form a healthy food habit now. It'll be easy for you because you've understood the significance and seen a live example. I will help you train your son to eat healthy.'

'Thank you, Meera, and thank you so much, Samyukta dear! You are really an angel!'

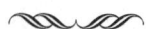

Sahana: Aunty, it really sounds wise and easy to condition the baby for healthy food habits in the womb.

Doctor: A stitch in time saves nine. I feel so upset when I see a two or three-year-old child eating chips and snacks from packets. The preservatives, colouring and flavouring agents are not good for health.

Fast foods are easy to eat but it's difficult for the body to get rid of the toxins. Also sugar, refined flour and processed food serve as 'fertilizer' for pathogenic bacteria (harmful) and yeast, causing them to rapidly multiply. Pathogenic bacteria cause inflammation of gut—resulting in allergy, infections, obesity, BP, diabetes, anxiety and depression. Junk food = high inflammation = poor gut health = poor immunity (low resistance to infections). Beneficial bacteria help in absorption, vitamin formation, hormone balance, weight reduction and optimal mental health.

Sahana: Aunty, are you against taking junk food?

Doctor: I won't be very stubborn in this, Sahana. We can have junk food occasionally. My advice is to try to enjoy whatever we eat, and not to feel guilty about it. To eat judiciously and not binge. One must set one's own limits in eating. Once in a while it's okay if you break it. Try to catch up later. Take plenty of water and fibre and do more exercise on that day. When we eat lovingly, guilt disappears, and nutrients are absorbed better.

Let's see what Dr Partha Nandhi, famous gastroenterologist in the US has to say:

'If you are in overall good health, I recommend following an 80/20 diet lifestyle. Eighty per cent of the time, you should be focused on healthy, real, unboxed/unprocessed foods. The rest of the time, you can have a little treat or something not as healthy. This ensures you are getting good nutrition to keep your body in optimum health while also enjoying yourself once in a while and indulging in your favourite treats.'[*]

Chef Manjit Singh Gill, president of the Indian Federation of Culinary Associations, says, 'You have to have a romantic relationship with food. Any food

---

[*] Nandi, Partha. *Ask Dr Nandi: 5 Steps to Becoming Your Own #HealthHero for Longevity, Well-Being, and a Joyful Life* (Delhi: Simon & Schuster, 2017).

and any quantity, when eaten with love, is good for the body. Thinking that food can make you fat is absurd. Stress, mental worries and sedentary lifestyle are some of the reasons behind obesity. When you are getting food and you are able to eat it, feel blessed."

Sahana: I understand that apart from food, our feelings are important. Aunty, how does one ensure happiness while eating healthy?

Doctor: The simple act of eating raises our levels of endorphins (happy hormone). This results in increased digestion, assimilation, and ultimately greater efficiency in calorie-burning. So happy eating doesn't cause obesity. When there is stress, cortisol is released, which desensitizes us to pleasure. We need to eat more food to feel the same amount of pleasure when we're stressed. This means that if you're anxious about gaining weight or frightened to eat a dessert, you'll generate more cortisol. Cortisol results in weight gain.

Sahana: Oh! Now I understand why some people gain weight in spite of eating less and why some don't gain weight in spite of eating more. The key is their feeling.

Doctor: I'm glad the point is well taken. Let's see the relationship between feelings and food.

Feelings and Food

Food serves a greater purpose than just appeasing the hunger in humans. It serves as happiness, comfort, luxury, celebration and, in many cases, even as security.

---

* Gill, Manjit. *Eating Wisely & Well* (Delhi: Penguin Books, 1997).

Some foods are identified with some regions—pickles in Andhra, coconut oil cooking in Kerala, fish in West Bengal, roti in north India and idly in Tamil Nadu. Food preferences are deeply ingrained in some cultures. That is why some people can't survive outside their region without their favourite food item, as they feel their identity and survival are threatened without it. Whenever humans gather to celebrate or relax, they prefer eating. There are two dimensions of eating: eating for health and eating for emotional upheavals, both positive and negative. Some eat to live and some live to eat. Food is associated with positive feelings of happiness and love, and negative feelings of guilt, craving and aversion.

Food and love on taste

Food that we believe has been prepared with tender loving care always tastes better. A study has shown that food we perceive to have been made with love tastes better. Two groups of people were invited to Christmas dinner. The first group were told that the food had been prepared in a traditional way with a lot of care and love. The second group was informed that the food was routinely prepared without much effort. All the first group people said the taste of the food was extraordinary. The results suggest that our emotional perception of taste can be enhanced or diminished by the amount of time, love and care that goes into meals, which ultimately can increase our enjoyment of food.* We feel convinced that nothing can beat our mother's biryani or grandmother's laddus. Japanese Tea Ceremony is an example of it. The Japanese tea ceremony is called Chanoyu, Sado or simply Ocha in Japanese. Preparing tea in this ceremony means pouring all one's attention into the predefined movements. The whole process is not about drinking tea, but is about aesthetics, preparing a bowl of tea with one's heart. Serving tea is an art and a spiritual discipline. Food and emotions are thus intertwined.

Dr Verny says, 'Eating is as much an emotional act for an infant as it is a physical one. Mother should eat with happiness and satisfaction. Babies in the womb are so sensitive to the food consumed by the mother that they will let the mother feel what makes him or her happy about the food eaten by the mother. It is like, more than the umbilical cord, it is the heart and feelings of the mother and the baby in her womb that are connected by an invisible but special cord. A pregnant mother should eat with all the love for herself and her baby in her womb. When served with love and care, the baby gets the best of nourishments in the womb.'†

Dr Deepak Chopra says, 'Paying attention to flavours, aromas, and colour in the diet will ensure that you are ingesting the foods you need in order to

---

* Taylors, Audrey. 'Science-backed Reasons Why Food Cooked with Love Is More Delicious', University Herald (7 December 2016), https://www.universityherald.com/articles/53686/20161207/science-backed-reasons-why-food-cooked-love-more-delicious.htm, accessed on 21 August 2025.
† Verny with Kelly. *The Secret Life*, 1981.

create a healthy body for you and your unborn baby. By paying attention to the tastes and colours, the diet will be delicious and nutritionally complete.

The process of creating a body from food is miraculous. You digest, absorb and metabolize the energy and information of your food into the intelligence of your body. Simultaneously, your unborn baby extracts and metabolizes the nutritional information in your bloodstream into his developing body.'*

Food can influence our mood depending on its content. Food can be a mood stressor or a mood supporter.

Foods behind That Latent Feeling of Depression

Food not only quenches physiological sensation of hunger but can profoundly influence psychological and mental state of mind. It has been proven beyond doubt that food can affect mood and the way we think. If you are depressed or anxiety-prone, your food habits could be the reason and it may actually be triggering it.

Mood Stressors

Sugar, caffeine, MSG (Monosodium Glutamate), artificial sweeteners, HFCS (High Fructose Corn Syrup), processed foods, alcohol etc., all affect mood and cause upheaval in the inner emotional systems.

---

* Chopra, *Magical Beginnings*, p. 74.

Reasons for Mood Swings

A lot of factors can throw the mood out of balance. 1) stress 2) hormonal imbalance 3) big shifts in blood sugar. Fluctuations in blood sugar levels cause mood variations. Low blood sugar can cause us to feel nervous or anxious and confused, while high blood sugar causes fatigue and worsens depression.

Foods That Reduce Depression and Anxiety

A hygienic and well-planned diet along with lots of water every day is sure to give you a refreshing sensation all day long. Eat healthy to remain fresh and active.

Mood Supporters

Water, vegetables, fruits (bananas, berries and citrus fruits), fish, nuts (almonds and also peanuts or cashews), seeds (sunflower seeds, pumpkin seeds) etc., are all foods that help you maintain emotional balance.

GUILT

In our experience, we found that when the mother relishes the food she eats, the baby doesn't pose any problem taking food after birth. If the mother feels guilty or dislikes taking the food, the same feeling is passed on to the baby in some cases.

Once, an expecting mother came to me for a check-up and the husband was complaining that she was not taking food properly. When I started to advise, Mahita said vehemently, 'Why do none of you understand my plight. I am just not able to eat. I get irritated by your advice, which worsens my situation.'

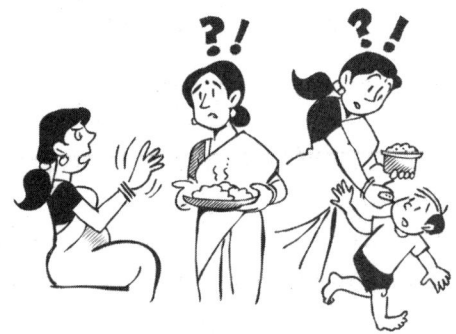

When expecting mom doesn't feel like eating, the same feeling is passed on to the baby.

I asked her not to bother about the advice and be herself and eat whatever she felt like eating and asked her husband not to force. In the next pregnancy, Mahita came to me in the ninth month and said, 'Doctor, you remember me? I got irritated by your advice on diet. I now understand the importance. This time I am eating well and eating with interest, because my first daughter doesn't eat at all. I see the exact replica of my feeling in her. It's such a great ordeal every day to feed her and it takes nearly two hours to make her eat.'

Sometimes the spouse or elders at home feel that the expecting mother is not taking sufficient food and keep complaining, 'You are not single now. You are not taking food properly. See, all the fruits are getting rotten. Responsible people do not waste food. Even if you don't take food for yourself, it's okay. You must eat at least for the sake of the baby.' This hurts many mothers. They feel, 'I'm not important to them; only the baby is important. Why should I eat?' Others start feeling guilty and blame themselves, 'What my mom or husband are saying must be true; I can't eat well.' With this guilty feeling, when they try to eat, they literally will not be able to relish food and end up eating less.

Suggestion to well-wishers:

They need to empathize with the expecting Mom by saying, 'See, in pregnancy, many women don't feel like taking food. It's ok *even* if you take less. But, do have a little. Take some more later. Try taking it in different ways and combinations. Frequent, small meals will give you some energy and you won't feel tired. Don't worry about wastage of food.

We need to remember that during pregnancy, even the bravest woman feels anxious and gets upset over a piece of good advice. She needs more pampering and moral support and that's the right way.

CRAVING

When people feel depressed, they crave various kinds of foods. It is this comfort and consolation eating that leads to weight gain.

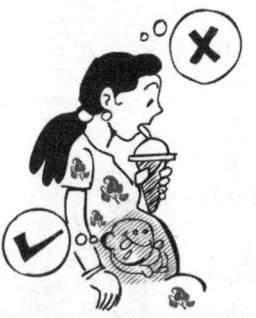
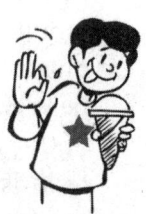

Sometimes the baby's wish is expressed as the mother's craving

Sometimes, thinking of an alternative, like listening to music, talking to a friend, walking or napping can also help deal with the cravings. Sometimes, when there is craving for chocolate, all that the pregnant mother needs is, more than anything else, a hug or a pat. It is often that we largely mistake the body's signals. Sometimes the wish of the unborn baby is expressed *Sometimes, baby's wish is expressed as craving of the expecting mom.* In some cases, it is observed that during pregnancy, mothers crave food items they didn't like before pregnancy. It may be the baby's wish being expressed through the mother. In such cases, it is observed that the baby likes the same food item after birth, and the mother goes back to her original food preference of not liking it.

Research on nutrition during pregnancy throws light on two important points: the quantity and long-term impact on the baby.

'Expecting Mother Should Eat for Two'

Mother need not literally eat for two (adult two). The quantity need not be very high. (Only 300 kcal more food is enough). If the mother takes nutritious food, it is sufficient for the unborn baby because of effective bio-utilization occurring during pregnancy.

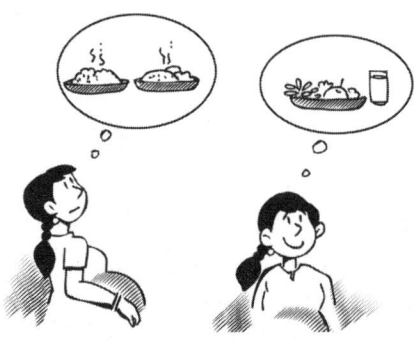

The expecting mom need not eat for two, having a nutritious and balanced diet is enough

1) The food she eats has an impact on her baby and the grandchild.

The food taken by the mother during pregnancy not only influences the baby she is carrying, but also her grandchild. We can understand when the mother is underfed during pregnancy (such as during famine), the baby has low birth weight. Research shows even the grandchild is born with less weight.

After the Dutch famine of 1944–45 (Hunger winter), towards the end of the Second World War in the Netherlands, the children of women who were pregnant were smaller than expected. However, when these children grew up and had children, those children also had low birth weight. Studies suggest that the damage suffered in early life leads to permanent impairment and might also affect the future generations. Its prevention will probably bring about important health, educational and economic benefits.[*] So, the mother has to take adequate, nutritious diet during pregnancy.

Regarding intake of food, we need to know two things. What to eat and how to eat.

What to Eat?

- The pregnancy diet ideally should be fresh, nutritious, easily digestible and rich in protein, iron, minerals and vitamins.

---

[*] Victora, Cesar G., et al. 'Maternal and child undernutrition: consequences for adult health and human capital', *The Lancet*, Vol. 371, no. 9609, pp. 340–357.

- Preference must be given to including natural foods in the diet rather than processed foods.
- Processed food is easy for one to eat but difficult for the body to process. It has been established that the body absorbs more energy from natural sources of food. To best explain with an analogy, one can observe the difference in the health and growth of plants that are watered every day with tap or well water versus rainwater.

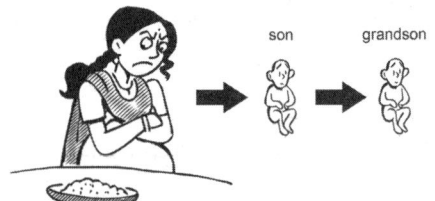

When the mother is underfed, the baby is born with low weight. This effect may be passed down to her grandchildren, too.

The most important nutrients required per day during pregnancy are:

1. Iron, 30–60 mg
2. Calcium, 1000 mg
3. Protein, 60 gm
4. Folic acid, 600–800 μg
5. Omega 3, 300 mg

They have to be taken in diet, apart from supplements.

Iron

Increases oxygen-carrying capacity in blood. Lack of iron is called anaemia, and it affects the mother and the baby. It causes weakness, increases susceptibility to infections, decrease in pain-bearing capacity and causes decrease in lactation and increase in puerperal sepsis in mother. It can also cause low birth weight in baby and preterm birth.

Iron is of two types: heme iron, which is an animal source and non-heme iron, which is a vegetarian source. Heme iron can be found in red meat, egg and fish. Non-Heme iron can be found in vegetables, green leafy vegetables, spinach, beans, peas, carrot, beetroot, tomato, potato, broccoli and lentils. Also in fruits such as strawberry, apple, pear, peach and plum. Iron-boosting fruits include citrus, melons and guava. Among dry fruits, iron can be found in dates, figs and raisins, and in seeds in almond, cashew, sunflower seeds, and pumpkin seeds. Take jaggery and use iron utensils for cooking. There are some studies that show the important link between improving health and enjoying what you eat.

In an unusual study, researchers from Sweden and Thailand joined forces to determine how cultural preferences for food affect the absorption of iron from a meal.[*] A group of women from each country was fed a typical Thai meal: rice, veggies, coconut, fish sauce and hot chilli paste. As fate would have it, Thai women enjoy Thai food but Swedish women don't. This proved to be a crucial metabolic fact, because, even though all the meals contained exactly the same amount of iron, the Swedish women absorbed only half as much as the Thai women. To complete this phase of the study, both groups received a typical Swedish

---

[*] David, Marc. 'The Pleasure of Eating and Its Metabolic Power', Psychology of Eating (13 February 2025), https://psychologyofeating.com/metabolic-power-pleasure/, accessed on 21 August 2025.

meal—hamburger, mashed potatoes, and string beans with exactly the same iron content. Not surprisingly, the Thai Women absorbed significantly less iron from their Swedish meal.

Next, the Thai women were separated into two groups. One group received the aforementioned Thai meal and the other was given the same exact meal as well, but that meal was first placed in a blender and turned to mush. Just imagine your favourite evening meal all whipped together into baby food. Once again, the same results were seen for their Swedish counterparts who had their Swedish meal turned into a frappe. The inescapable conclusion is that the nutritional value of a food is not merely given in the nutrients it contains, but is dependent upon the synergistic factors that help us absorb those nutrients. Remove Vitamin P: Pleasure, and the nutritional value of our food plummets.

We had observed the impact of faith and anxiety on iron absorption during pregnancy.

For Lakshmi, it was her first pregnancy and she was coming for a check-up from the sixth month. Her haemoglobin was nine grams and I put her on iron tablets and put her on an anaemia diet. After one month, when the haemoglobin didn't increase, she became anxious. She said she was taking medicines without fail and also the prescribed diet regularly and still HB was not improving. I changed the iron tablet and asked her to take it two hours after food and reassured her that next month the haemoglobin would improve.

Around that time, another pregnant mother from a village was also coming for an antenatal checkup;

she has been married for ten years and conceived after taking fertility treatment with us. Her haemoglobin was seven grams in the sixth month. I told her to take medicines regularly and explained the diet in detail and warned her about the consequences of anaemia. No sooner did I finish my sermon, she replied in a confident tone 'Amma, in my village, I don't get any of the food items you suggested. I can take only one glass of milk every day; you give medicines with your own hands, I will take the tablets regularly and then my blood will certainly improve'. I was surprised by her audacity. When she came after one month, her haemoglobin had gone up to nine grams and I was amazed at the power of faith. The town patient came one month later, and her haemoglobin was again nine grams. It was not improving; this time her mother-in-law had come with her and she was more anxious and was asking whether blood transfusion was necessary. I told her that injectable iron would suffice. When her mother-in-law was repeatedly asking about blood transfusion, I asked her why she was keen about it and told her that Lakshmi's condition didn't warrant blood transfusion. She said that her eldest daughter-in-law had had blood transfusion during pregnancy and so she was worried whether Lakshmi would also need it. This worry was unconsciously passed on to Lakshmi, which was preventing her haemoglobin from increasing, despite regularly taking medicines and following proper diet. When the mother-in-law's doubt was cleared, Lakshmi's haemoglobin count rose to ten grams next month. Anxiety or confidence can be easily passed on from a person of authority, esteem and intimacy. Anxiety prevents the success of treatment while faith and confidence ensure success.

Calcium

Helps in building bones and teeth of the baby.

Sources:

- Milk: 300 mg/cup
- Yoghurt: 370 mg/cup
- Cottage Cheese: 138 mg/cup
- Sesame Seeds: 200 mg/tablespoon
- Spinach: 250 mg
- Cabbage, cauliflower, broccoli, orange: 60 mg
- Dates: 15 mg
- Almond, figs, raisins

Absorption is increased by vitamin D and magnesium and is decreased by salt, coffee, alcohol, phytates (nuts and grains) and oxalates in spinach.

Protein

Building block of tissues.

- Milk: 8 g/cup
- Curd: 10 g/cup
- Cheese: 14 g/cup

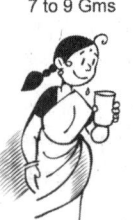

7 to 9 Gms

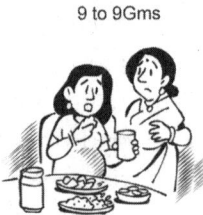

9 to 9Gms

- Lentil: 15 g/cup
- Beans: 18 gm/cup
- Nuts and seeds
- Egg: 6 g
- Chicken: 27 g (1/2 roasted chicken breast)
- Fish: 23 g/3 ounces

Folic Acid

It prevents:

1) Neural tube defect
2) Recurrent miscarriages
3) Pre-eclampsia
4) Low birth weight

Sources: Lentils, spinach and orange

Omega-3 Fatty Acid—DHA 300 mg

Effect on foetus:

1) Brain and eye development
2) Decreases prematurity and low birth weight
3) Allergy and eczema

On mother: Decreases pre-eclampsia and depression

Sources: Flaxseed, walnut, cold-water fatty fish (salmon, sardine, cod, halibut)

Tips on How to Eat

- Mothers must practise eating with awareness. Choose at least one meal a week to eat in silence, noticing the flavours, sensations and aromas that nurture us.
- Eat meals in a peaceful and settled environment.
- Enjoy eating with friends and relatives.

Advantages of sitting on the floor while eating: It improves digestion, helps to reduce weight, improves the posture, makes us more flexible, lubricates and keeps knee and hip joints healthy, relaxes the mind and calms the nerves and strengthens the heart by improving circulation.

Chew soft food well, five to ten times and dense food fifteen to twenty times before swallowing it. Sit quietly for a few minutes after finishing the meal. Mother who practises 'Talking to the Baby in the Womb' during pregnancy can tell the baby just before eating, 'I'm eating for you, so you'll be healthy and happy.' This strengthens the mother–baby bonding. Experiments have proved that the baby in the womb is actually capable of enjoying the food mother eats and can retain the taste preference even after birth. Here are some of the great benefits of family meals, according to research reviewed by Martha Marino and Sue Butkus of Washington State University.

Benefits of Family Meals

- Kids' thinking skills and linguistic development improve. (This may be due to the longer

conversations that tend to take place during family meals.)
- Family meals contribute to a child's healthy development even more than play or story time.
- Teens who eat more meals with their families are less likely to be depressed.
- Teens who share more family meals experience better relationships with their families and friends.

Case of Madhuri: How Talking to the Baby in the Womb Is Effective in Ensuring Health of the Baby

Madhuri was a working woman and conceived while preparing for a competitive exam. She was too busy with her work and exam preparation, it seemed she hardly ever remembered she was carrying. Her mother-in-law kept on worrying, 'If you don't take proper food now, how will be the baby?' Madhuri was practising Talking to the Baby in the Womb very well. She used to tell her baby, 'Though I love you with all my heart, I can't spend much time with you. Please understand my position and cooperate with me'. Before eating she used to say 'All that I'm eating, should reach you. I want you to be healthy and

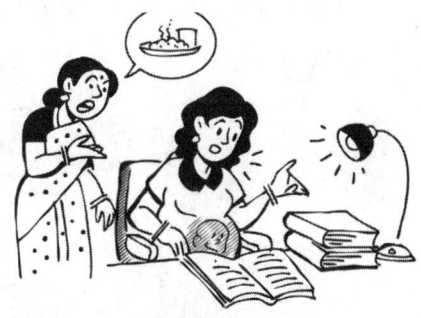

If you don't eat properly now, how will the baby be?

happy.' The baby used to respond through movements and she was relaxed because her baby's support was there for her.

She had a very easy normal delivery and to the surprise of her mother-in law, the baby was healthy and weighed 3 kg. So, it is not what we eat; the intention also matters.

Don'ts while Eating

- Don't overeat; leave about a third of the stomach empty to aid digestion
- Avoid eating when you are upset.
- While eating, don't watch television, read books, messages, talk over cell phone, etc.

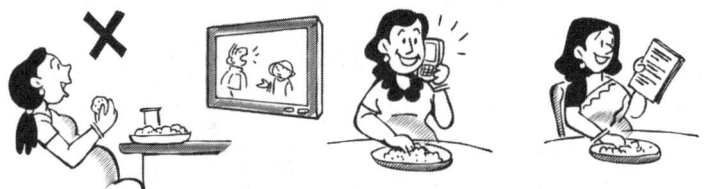

Left side: Don't watch TV while eating
Right side: Don't talk or read while eating

Mythology

Once Lord Krishna got a message that sage Durvasa was going to stay in his palace as a guest. Lord Krishna took all precautions to keep the sage happy, as he was known for his short temper—he would utter a curse even for a minor breach of discipline. As part of the preparation, Lord Krishna instructed his cook to make extra efforts to provide sumptuous and delicious meals so that the sage would not be displeased. The cook promised to do his best. Sage Durvasa relished all the dishes and was overjoyed. Later, when Lord Krishna asked the cook about how he had managed to please the sage, the cook replied that he had learnt from Durvasa's mother the sage's favourite dishes. He had prepared all of them and so the sage felt as if he had tasted his mother's preparation.

Doctor: Sahana, it's said that exercise is like a king and nutrition a queen. When we combine the two, we get the kingdom of health.

Sahana: That's a wonderful quote, Aunty. Thanks for enlightening me about pregnancy diet and my attitude towards food. I understand the importance of eating the right food and eating it with love and care, as it can affect the next two generations. As you shared about the secrets of mother's food tasting better, I have made up my mind to prepare healthy and tasty food for my baby and make sure he or she enjoys every bit of it. Are there any other tips to make my baby healthy? Because I see some children who keep catching cold, cough and fever frequently.

Doctor: Mother who needs to improve her immunity, must take healthy diet, regular exercise, adequate sleep and good relationships—all these are part of a holistic approach to boosting the immune system and protecting from disease. There is an important thing to improve lifelong immunity of the baby. Can you guess what it is?

Sahana: Any clues, Grandma?

Lakshmi Aunty: In our days we never took any pill for ourselves or for the baby, we only breast fed the baby; our babies were healthy—no cough, cold or any fever.

Doctor: Wow! Lakshmi aunty, you said it! Yes! It's mother's milk. Mother's milk is indeed nature's life-giving elixir to the baby.

Sahana: Aunty, please enlighten me on breastfeeding?

The milk produced soon after delivery is called colostrum, it is very nutritious; mothers must start breast feeding within one hour of birth. This helps in ensuring continuation of breast feeding. Milk produced later is called mature milk.

The mature milk consists of

1. Fore milk
2. Hind milk

Fore Milk comes from the start of the feed; it's watery and satisfies the baby's thirst. Hind milk comes later in a feed, is richer in fat, gives energy and lowers hunger.

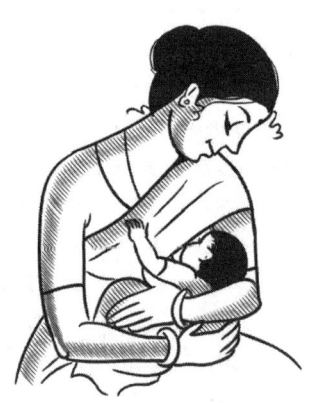

Nutrition and Diet

Health benefits of breast milk:

- Breast feeding enhances brain development and increases IQ by eight points.
- Breastfed babies are less prone to respiratory infections, diarrhoea, urinary infections, ear infections, etc.
- Breastfed babies are less prone to obesity, diabetes, heart diseases, eczema, asthma and other allergic disorders later in life.

Sahana: How to ensure an adequate supply of milk, Aunty?

Doctor: Mother must have strong intention to feed the baby (because breast feeding is hormone dependent) and take adequate diet and rest. She has to feed the baby frequently with proper positioning of the baby.

Sahana: Aunty, are there any special food items to increase milk production?

Doctor: Lakshmi aunty, you may be knowing more about it, please share with us.

Lakshmi aunty: Green leafy vegetables, carrot, beetroot, bottle gourd, drumstick, raw papaya and bitter gourd; watermelon, almond; fenugreek, fennel, cumin, garlic; bread, oats, rice and fish, bajra, plenty of water, milk; and confidence of mother and moral support of family. This is all I know.

Sahana: Grandma. I never knew that you knew so much. I'll surely take your advice. Thank you so much, Aunty. Your experiences and explanations have cleared all my doubts.

Doctor: God bless you, dear, with a wonderful child. Happy pregnancy and happy, easy and safe normal delivery. Please remember our primary goal must be a healthy and happy child; the mode of delivery is secondary. In case a Caesarean section is warranted, we must accept it wholeheartedly. After a month, no one will remember anything about the type of delivery. Sahana, my journey with you, juggling the memory, has made me feel enriched and rejuvenated.

Sahana: I sincerely thank you, Aunty, from the bottom of my heart, for the clarity and understanding of the concept of Talking to the Baby in the Womb and its influence on various aspects of pregnancy and beyond. I'll practise Talking to the Baby in the Womb and join hands with you in spreading it to others.

Nutrition and Diet

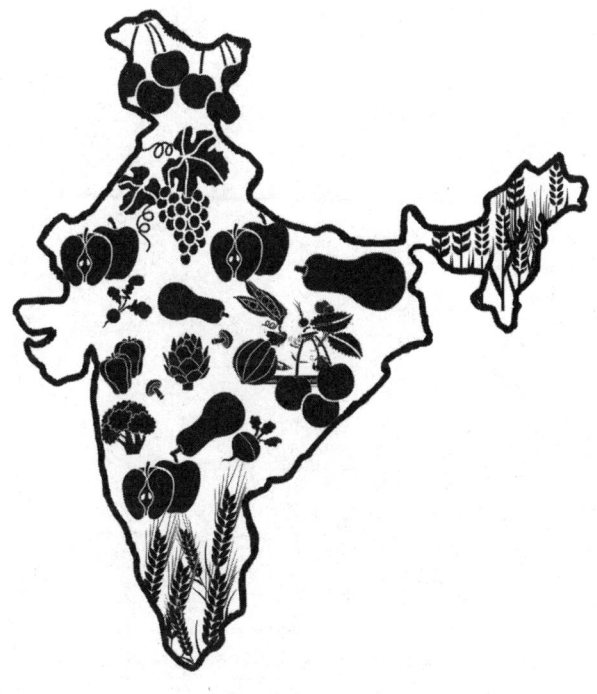

'The doctor of the future will no longer treat the human frame with drugs, but rather will cure and prevent diseases with nutrition.'

—Thomas A. Edison

Acknowledgements

At the outset, I would like to thank my 'obstetrician', who helped me conceive and 'deliver' this book, my brother, Ashok, who pushed me into this project, guided and patiently waited for the birth of this book.

My heartfelt thanks to all the mothers and their families whose experiences form the content of this book.

I sincerely thank my colleagues Madhavi, who worked as my right hand in the preparation of this script, Dr Hazira, Dr Aruna Kumari, Dr Nirupama, Dr Prameela, Dr Jyothi and Mrs Deepa, who helped me in compiling and supervision.

Special thanks to our close family friend Prof. Raghurama Raju, without whose help and guidance this book would not have seen the light of the world.

Special thanks to Miss Deepa Ramakrishnan for patiently going through the script and helping to bring out this book.

Also thanks to Mr Gopinath, a motivational speaker, and Dr Nalinikanth, who is a behavioural scientist and motivational speaker.

I remember with gratitude my friends Sudha Mohan and Sudha Prasanna, who sat with me for long hours at odd times for discussion and correction of the material. Well-wishers Girija, Dr Sathyapriya, Dr Obul Reddy and brother-in-law Ravindra gave me strong moral support.

My husband, Dr Bhaskar, who is the mastermind behind our show, as usual offered solid rock-like support with his insight and planning. Our staff, who are like family, adjusted to my erratic work schedule remarkably. My daughter, Dr Divya and son-in-law Dr Bala Sundaram for their love and moral support.

My special thanks to Rajesh Raghunathan, who, in spite of his busy schedule, came to my hospital from a far-off place and spent many days discussing and writing the script. He got so involved in this project that he could translate this book into Tamil with amazing ease.

I express my deep gratitude to Pillai for his unique contribution of life-like cartoons.

I thank my brothers and sisters-in-law, Dr Rajkumar and Sujatha, Ashok and Malathi, Ranganathan and Thenmozhi, Kumaravel and Veena and sisters Vijayalakshmi and Ramanishankar, nephews and nieces and Kishore Menon for sharing their views, and for their advice and encouragement.

I am inspired by the pioneering works of Dr Deepak Chopra, Dr Thomas Verny, Dr Bruce

Lipton and Dr Chamberlain, and I have quoted them at appropriate places and I remember them with gratitude.

My *pranams* to my parents, parents-in-law, grandparents, who have been a guiding light in my everyday life. I have no words that can adequately express my gratitude to god and my gurus for their constant blessings and guidance.

Annexure

FAQs

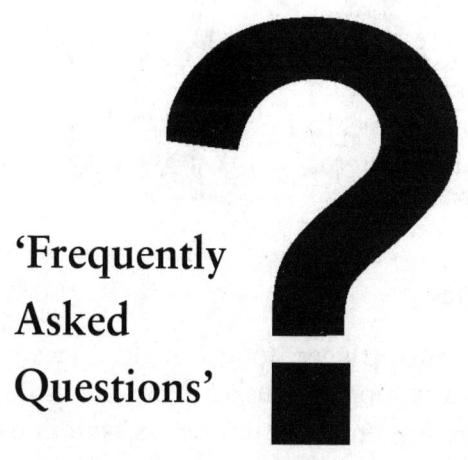

'Frequently Asked Questions'

Annexure

Though pregnancy is a natural function, when a problem arises, there may be risk to the mother and the baby. That's why pregnancy check-up is necessary to detect and manage problems, when they arise, because every pregnancy must culminate in the birth of a healthy baby and healthy mother. These guidelines are general information and the expectant mother has to clear her specific doubts personally with the treating doctor.

1) HEARTBURN IN PREGNANCY:

a) Relaxation of Lower Oesophageal Sphincter (LES) in lying position and after a heavy meal.
b) The growing uterus presses on the stomach.

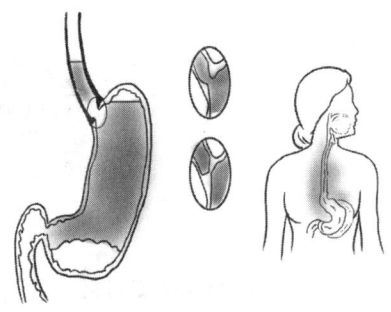

Control Measures:

- Avoid heartburn-trigger foods, highly seasoned spicy food, fatty foods, citrus, caffeine and alcohol.
- Break it up: six small meals are the solution to heartburn, bloating and lagging energy level.
- Rituals of eating: sit upright while eating—stay that way for a couple of hours after you eat.
- Chew it over: Chewing is the first step in the digestive process. When we eat fast, we swallow air-forming gas pockets in the belly.

- Do not drink too much water while you're eating, this will distend the stomach, aggravating heartburn.
- Have a meal at least two hours before bedtime.
- Lying down, slouching, slumping, and stooping will increase it.
- And when you have to bend, do it with your knees instead of at your waist.
- Prop with pillows: Try sleeping with your head elevated about six inches.
- Loose and comfortable clothes: wear loose clothes.
- Tight clothes aggravate it.

Solutions:

- Chew sugarless gum after meals: It helps reduce excess acid.
  A tablespoon of honey in warm milk (low-fat skim milk) can be yummy and relaxing.
- Medicines: Antacids, PPI, H2 receptor blockers.

2) CONSTIPATION

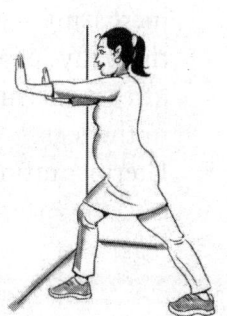

1. Constipation is one of the common symptoms that occur during pregnancy. Generally we need more fibre in the diet along with liquids and good intestinal

motility to pass stool freely. During pregnancy, because of vomiting, there is lesser intake of diet and more fluid loss. Due to pregnancy hormone (progesterone), intestinal motility will be sluggish. So to come out of this complaint, we have to take a more fibre-rich diet, more water and do walking.

2. It is related to emotional status also. As anus is a sphincter, when we are mentally free, sphincter opens and products are emptied. We can see that we pass freely in the toilet at our house and can't pass freely in a toilet in an unfamiliar place.

SUGGESTIONS:

Take plenty of fluids, add more fibre in the form of plenty of green leafy vegetables, fruits like banana, apple, guava and raisins. Chew well.

Medicine: Digestive enzyme, magnesium and laxative when necessary.

3) LEG CRAMPS: Third trimester, late night CAUSES:

- Muscles strain due to increasing weight of the baby, progesterone, affects the muscle tone in the legs.
- Uterus putting pressure on the veins in the legs.

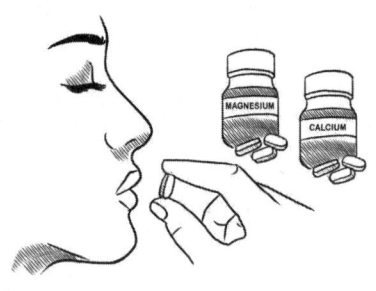

- Nutrients and salts, such as calcium or magnesium deficiency.
- Is there anything we can do to prevent leg cramps?
- Calf stretches: Stand a metre from a wall and lean forwards with arms outstretched to touch the wall. Keep the soles of your feet flat on the floor. Hold for five seconds. Repeat.
- Exercise for five minutes, three times a day, especially before going to bed.
- Daily foot exercises: Bend and stretch each foot up and down thirty times. Then rotate each foot eight times one way and eight times the other way.
- Try not to stand for long periods or sit with your legs crossed.
- At night-time, have a warm bath before going to bed.
- Try raising your feet on a pillow, or raise the foot not higher than 20 cm.
- Calcium and magnesium supplement.

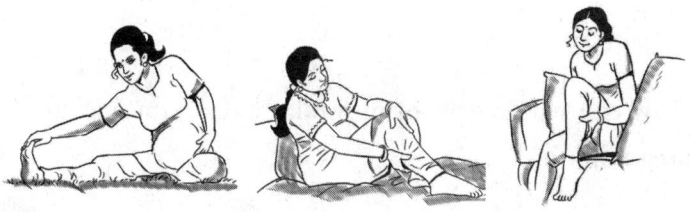

What to do during leg cramps?

- Flex your foot (extend your heel and point your toes toward your head). It may hurt at first, but the pain will gradually go away.

4) BACK PAIN DURING PREGNANCY:

- Massage the muscle.
- Get out of bed and walk around for a few minutes.

- Hormones released during pregnancy allow ligaments in the pelvic area to soften and the joints to become looser that may affect the support that the back normally experiences.

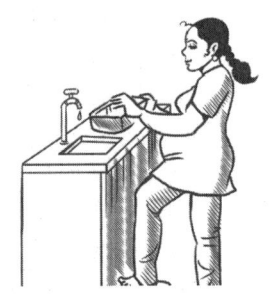

- Additional weight of pregnancy.
- Centre of gravity, which causes our posture to change.
- Poor posture, excessive standing, and bending can trigger or escalate the pain you experience in your back.

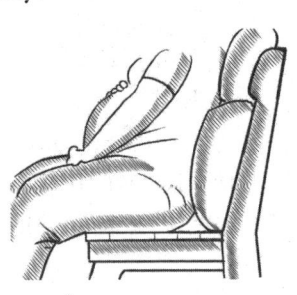

How can we prevent or minimize back pain during pregnancy?

- Avoid high heels and other shoes that do not provide adequate support.
- Squat to pick up something instead of bending over.

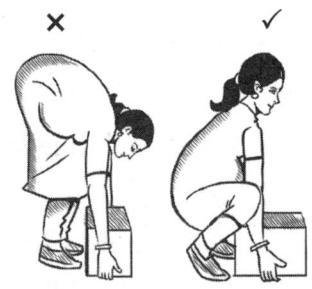

- Avoid sleeping on back. Sleep on side, and use a support pillow under your knees.
- Get plenty of rest.
- Exercises approved by healthcare provider.
- Consider consulting an orthopaedic.

POSTURES AND EXERCISES TO PREVENT BACK PAIN: Cat–Cow Exercise

Cow Pose 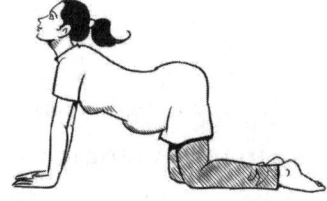   Cat Pose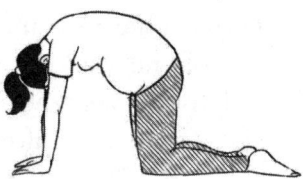

5) WHAT IS SLEEP HYGIENE?

Sleep hygiene is defined as behaviours that one can do to help promote good sleep using behavioural interventions.

Sleep hygiene tips:

- Maintain a regular sleep routine. Go to bed at the same time. Wake up at the same time.
- Avoid or minimize coffee, tea, soda, cigarettes, alcohol; it's best to limit coffee to early afternoon at the latest.

- Exercise regularly. Stop exercising four hours before sleep.

SLEEP SANCTUARY

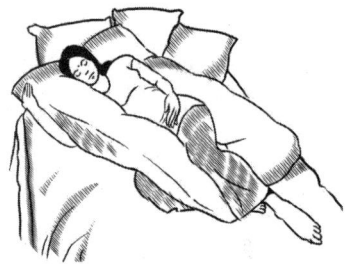

- Don't watch TV or read in bed.
- Watching TV or reading in bed, associate the bed with wakefulness; the bed is reserved for sleep.
- Turn off the TV, laptop, cell phone one hour before sleep. It suppresses melatonin (sleep hormone), causing delay in sleep.
- Have a quiet, comfortable bedroom. A little cooler and dark. Turn off bright lights.
- Have a comfortable mattress.
- A comfortable pre-bedtime routine.
- A warm bath, shower.
- Have a light snack—warm milk with honey, banana, walnuts, almond, peanut, cherry juice, etc.
- Meditation, or quiet time visualization, deep breathing, yoga, swing, chanting, soothing music, etc.
- Shoulder massage, and gentle head massage.
- Daytime sleep may be allowed for twenty to thirty minutes between 1.30–3 p.m.

If sleep is disturbed at night, just wake up and do some activity. Don't worry about sleep disturbance.

6) ARE JOURNEYS SAFE DURING PREGNANCY?

Journeys are safe in an uncomplicated pregnancy. In general, long journeys are best avoided in the first and third trimesters. Expecting mothers are advised not to undertake a journey when they have:

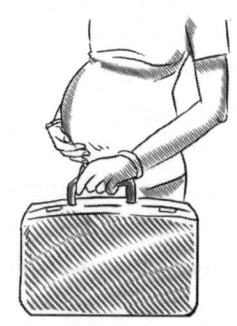

1. Twins, polyhydramnios (Excess amniotic fluid) and history of previous miscarriages.
2. With complaints of abdominal pain, bleeding per vagina, excess white discharge, urine infection etc.

Before undertaking long journeys, one must take the doctor's advice. In my experience, the fear and doubt instilled by others about journeys cause more harm. I have seen mothers take precautions, travel with conviction and confidence and not face any problem.

7) WHITE DISCHARGE: IS IT NORMAL OR ABNORMAL?

Normal white discharge is thin, milky with mild smell; it is harmless. White discharge due to infection causes discomfort like foul smell and itching; it may be yellow, greenish or

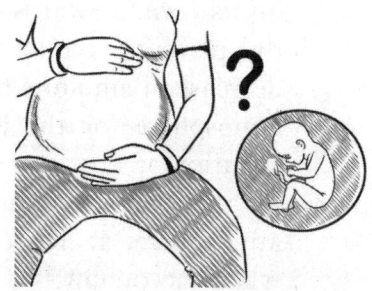

curdy white. Some infections may lead to miscarriage or premature labour. It must be treated.

White discharge of labour (delivery) will be jelly-like, and may be blood-stained. This white discharge indicates the opening of the cervix. It may be associated with back pain, tightness of the abdomen, pressure in lower abdomen or pelvis. Any white discharge excess in quantity or associated with other symptoms must be seen by a gynaecologist as early as possible.

8) WHAT IS THE IDEAL TIME FOR DELIVERY IN THE NINTH MONTH?

Usually, the time of delivery is determined by the baby.

1. The baby communicates to the mother's uterus when it is ready to take birth by sending signals in the form of hormones. This initiates labour. The delivery time varies from person to person. It may also vary in each delivery for the same mother.
2. The baby is said to be mature by thirty-seven weeks i.e., two weeks from the beginning of the ninth month. The baby will then be able to survive on its own. Towards the end of the ninth month, the placental blood flow decreases, resulting in decrease in amniotic fluid leading to unfavourable atmosphere for the baby in the womb. In that situation, it's better if the baby is delivered.
3. If the baby continues in an unfavourable atmosphere, it passes motion (meconium) and when meconium is aspirated, it causes problems

for the baby. This possibility is high in post-term pregnancy (after completion of ninth month).

Therefore, it is better to have frequent check-ups (weekly once) in the ninth month and visit doctor when there is decrease in foetal movement, pain in the abdomen, bleeding or leaking. Depending on the state of cervix, maturity and well-being of the baby, the doctor will decide whether to wait for spontaneous labour or induce it. It is alright for the baby to be delivered any time after the thirty-seventh week.

9) LEAKING

Leaking of amniotic fluid any time during pregnancy calls for immediate medical attention. Leaking in the seventh or eighth month is definitely a cause for concern, as it leads to premature labour and infection. Leaking in the ninth month helps initiation or augmentation of delivery. Leaking that occurs before the onset of labour pains requires induction of labour. Leaking that occurs after the onset of labour helps in the hastening of delivery.

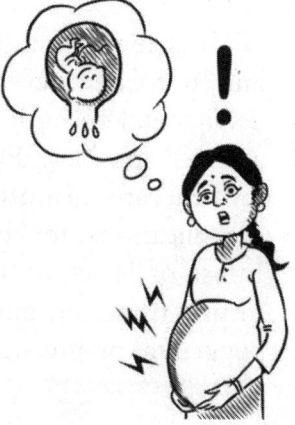

Hence, an expectant mother must be on the alert. She should be able to differentiate leaking from excessive white discharge and urine. When in doubt, it is better to see the doctor.

10) BLEEDING

Bleeding any time during the pregnancy is abnormal. Seeking immediate medical care is mandatory for maternal and foetal well being.

First and second trimester: Causes of bleeding could be sub-chorionic hematoma, cervical polyp, threatened miscarriage.

Precipitating factors: Physical strain, sexual contact, journey, urinary infections, infective white discharge, spicy food, etc.

Third trimester: APH (Antepartum Haemorrhage) and labour (delivery).

So, a pregnant woman must seek medical help and advice whenever there is bleeding.

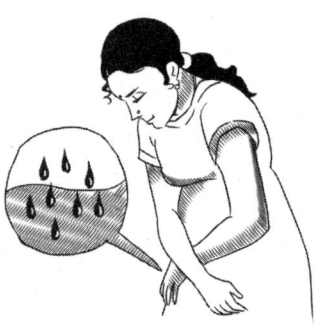

11) FEVER

Fever is an ominous symptom and untreated fever can be detrimental to both the baby and the mother. Emergency medical care is a must, to avoid complications for the baby. Effect of Fever on the baby: in first trimester: miscarriage; congenital malformation.

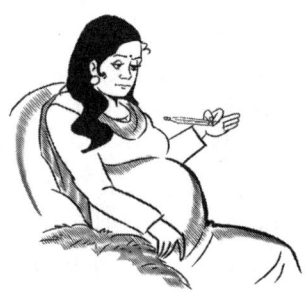

In the ninth month: Oligohydramnios (decrease amniotic fluid), meconium aspiration, risk to life etc.

Bleeding, leaking, excess white discharge, fever, pain in the abdomen are notorious symptoms. Hence, expecting mothers should not hesitate to report to the treating doctor as early as possible for evaluation and treatment.

Testimonials

Here are the personal experiences of some mothers who diligently followed the TALKING TO THE BABY IN THE WOMB technique and shared their experiences.

Mrs Swetha

This wonderful technique helped me to bond with the baby and experience motherhood right from the womb. I started talking to my baby from the ninth week of my pregnancy. Initially, I couldn't feel any movements. I talked to the baby about good books, my daily activities,

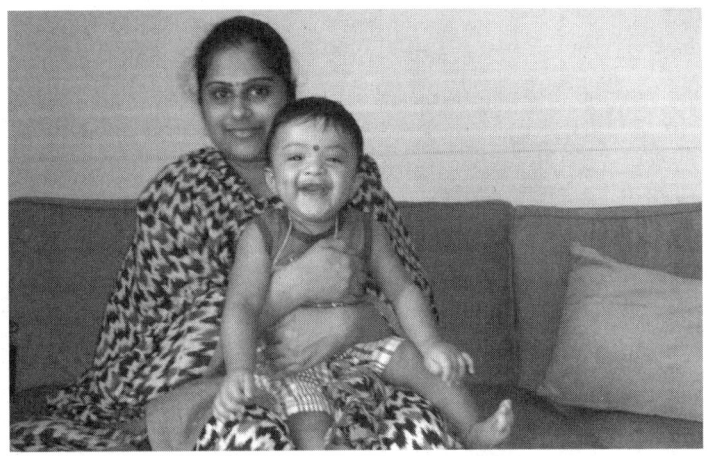

music and my dreams about him. Somewhere deep in my heart, I believed that my little one was listening to me and reciprocating in his own way.

Our First Meeting

My little one opened his eyes and gave me a big smile for the very first time. I called him by his name. He seemed to have recognized my voice and showed our special bond. He responded very well throughout the journey to his father's conversations. My brother had a special bond with him throughout my pregnancy as he was following up the test results and was talking with the baby regularly. When my brother came to see my little one, baby felt comfortable meeting him. While leaving, when my brother said 'Goodbye', he responded by waving his hand, indicating their special bond. This happened at their very first meeting. My baby stays calm and comfortable with his grandmother and never cries even if I am away. He acknowledges everything with a smile when I convey something. When I play a song, he feels comfortable and gestures as if he were familiar with that song. He became quiet the moment that song was played. That's the magic of the song.

In short, this technique helped me to know about my baby and build a strong bond of love. I feel I have known him for a longer period than his age. Besides me, everyone in my family felt the magic of Talking to the Baby in the womb and strongly believes in its power. Thanks a ton to my beloved Dr Andal Madam and Dr Bhaskar sir, who introduced this technique to me.

I admire Dr Andal for the great service she is doing in teaching mothers to bring an extraordinary generation of good children thereby building a better society.

I am a proud and happy mother to a lovable, intelligent and responsible child.

Mrs Ramani

My first baby had a mild ADHD problem. It was problematic to feed. As doctors said that baby might become normal in six years; he is normal now. I was afraid to have a second child. But now, as the doctors had indicated, he is normal. When I conceived a second time, I visited Dr Andal's Hospital in the fourth month of my pregnancy. Then Madam explained to me about 'Talking to the Baby in the womb' technique. Initially, I was not talking to my baby properly. But

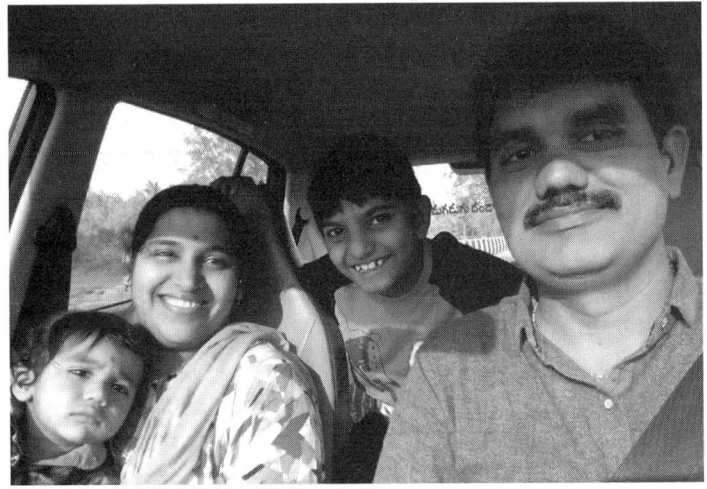

during the sixth month, I received my baby's kick for the first time. From that moment, I started believing 'Talking to the Baby in the womb' technique. I used to share every happy moment and sorrow with my baby. Similarly, my BP was not in control. It started rising. I practised 'Talking to the Baby in the womb' and brought it under control without medication.

I couldn't breast-feed my first baby. So, during my second pregnancy, I used to say to my baby, 'I should have enough milk for you after delivery, and you should drink only mother's milk.' For six months, he took only breast milk without any substitutes. Now, my baby is nine months old. He repeats all the words and sounds. He understands all my words. When he goes near the gas stove and I say, 'it will burn you', he comes back. We are carrying our baby on long journeys without any problem. All this has been possible only due to Dr Andal Bhaskar's 'Talking to the Baby in the womb' technique. I'll be eternally thankful to Dr Andal Ma'am and their staff.

I congratulate Dr Andal Bhaskar for inventing this technique of Talking to the Baby in the Womb and passing it on to all the pregnant mothers for building a good generation with peace, happiness and moral values.

Mrs Ankamma

My name is N. Venkateswaralu. I am working in DRDA at Sydapuram Mandal in Nellore district. I was married to Ankamma in 2012. We were told about Dr Andal's Talking to the baby in the Womb technique. From then on, I used to talk to my baby.

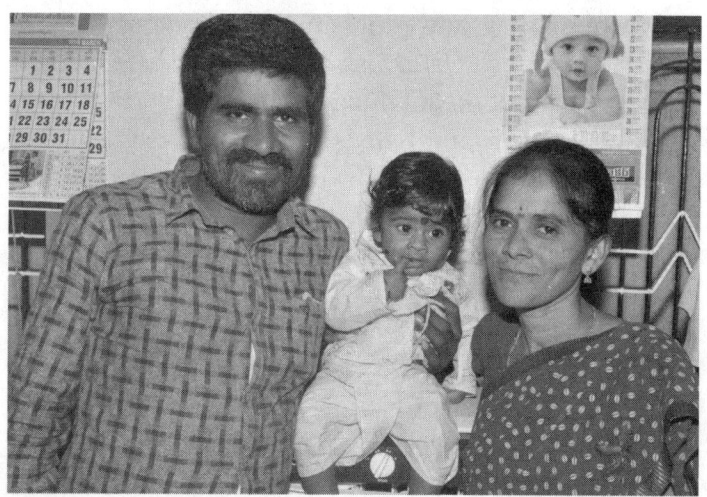

Every day at 9 a.m., while I was leaving for duty, Ankamma would tell the baby, 'Daddy is going to office, say "Bye" to him', he would immediately kick. When I was back home in the evening, my wife would say to the baby, 'Daddy has come back'. He would immediately give a kick. We used to say, 'I love you, Naanna. You are God's gift. We both like you very much, Naanna'. Every time when we said 'I love you Naanna', the baby used to give a quick response. Madam asked us to select any song and listen to it frequently as it was going to help Ankamma during her delivery and feeding time. We then selected a song from the movie 'Nani' and after he had got used to it, the baby slowly started responding to that song. During our talk with the baby, we used to say, 'You should have a good attitude towards others, you should go to a higher position in society'. He would respond by giving a kick. While talking to the baby, Ankamma used to say, 'You have to be delivered normally without any problem and labour pains have to start only when Daddy is with us because if Daddy is away, we cannot do anything individually'.

After delivery, on baby's sixth day, we wanted to check Talking to the baby in the womb technique. So, while he was being fed, we 'told' him to stop. He stopped drinking. Moments later we asked him to resume drinking milk, and he did! So, we understood that because of the Talking to the baby in the womb technique, the baby was recognizing our voice and responding to our words.

We congratulate Dr Andal for the effort in bringing out this Talking to the Baby technique and teaching us to have a good child. Thank you, Dr Andal Ma'am for giving us our wonderful baby.

Mrs Rajini Chinni

My journey with my baby started before I conceived. After my first son was born. I had three abortions for three consecutive years.

Andal Ma'am encouraged me to have a second baby, created faith in me by suggesting a few things. She insisted that I nourish myself with proper diet, a few yogic and breathing exercises. I was also given training in doing a few exercises in her hospital.

As advised by the doctors, I followed the above physical and mental steps. To my great surprise, I conceived exactly after three months.

It was at this time that Dr Andal advised me to talk to the baby in the womb. I followed each and every

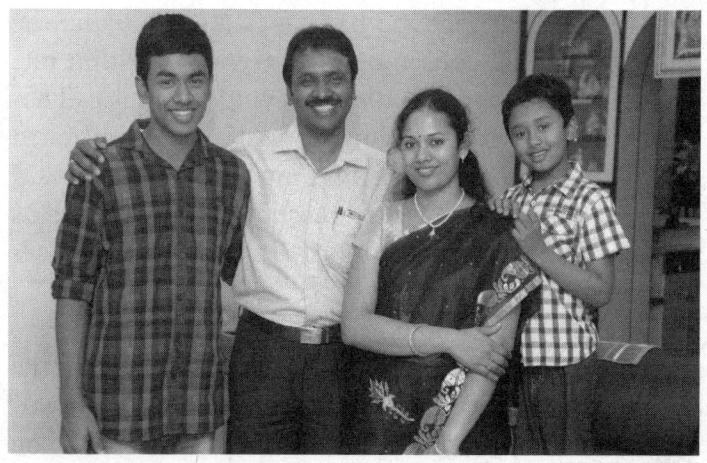

suggestion till my delivery. My journey was exciting and unforgettable. I was continuously interacting with the baby while reading books, watching TV, and when having my food. While eating, I used to think that every bite of this food was going to nourish my baby to become strong and healthy. This made me to choose healthy food throughout. I started imagining that my baby was growing healthier. I started reading books of my interest. That made me relax and helped solve many puzzles and improve my thinking powers. I learnt many new things and gained knowledge in the fields of my interest. I enjoyed many jokes too. Medical science says that when one is in happy mood, Serotonin, a feel-good hormone, is released. The small baby movements made me feel-good hormone, is released. The small baby movements made me feel that the baby is with me always. I listened to soothing music and songs that had a special appeal for me. Sometimes, when listening to particular songs again and again, I felt that the baby was also enjoying the music. I became conscious of movements within me. I felt that the baby was also enjoying the music. That indeed was a great feeling. On the TV I watched many funny programmes, and my favourite movies. I shunned things that created discomfort in my mind as I believed that every feeling of the mother influences the baby in the womb.

It is a fabulous and unforgettable journey that every mother goes through when the baby is growing in the womb. 'Talking to the Baby in the womb' is a way to interact with your baby. As the day progresses, you will notice its importance and start interacting more and more. As the delivery time approached, I got more excited. And I was sure that I would be blessed with a lovely baby. Finally I won. The baby was exactly as I had wished.

Yes! Talking to the baby in the womb is a powerful tool to connect with your baby, endowed with qualities you always wished to see in it.

I understood Dr Andal has discovered this technique of Talking to the Baby in the Womb by interacting with thousands of mothers, observing pregnant mothers and going through lot of literature regarding mother–baby bonding in pregnancy. What I felt extremely happy about my baby's response by movement to my thoughts, words and talk; it was a thrilling experience. I was astonished to learn that I could mould the personality of my baby in the womb. I understand the desire of Dr Andal that every mother in this world should practice this technique and bring in a generation of great people, such that all of us can live in peace and happiness. I appreciate what she is doing to pregnant mothers like me and it is a great service to the nation. I hope every pregnant mother does it and change the fate of this nation.

Thank you, Dr Andal for your guidance and encouragement.

Mrs Sridevi and Mr Dileep

The very first time you hold your baby, you may imagine it is a clean slate, unmarked by life. However,

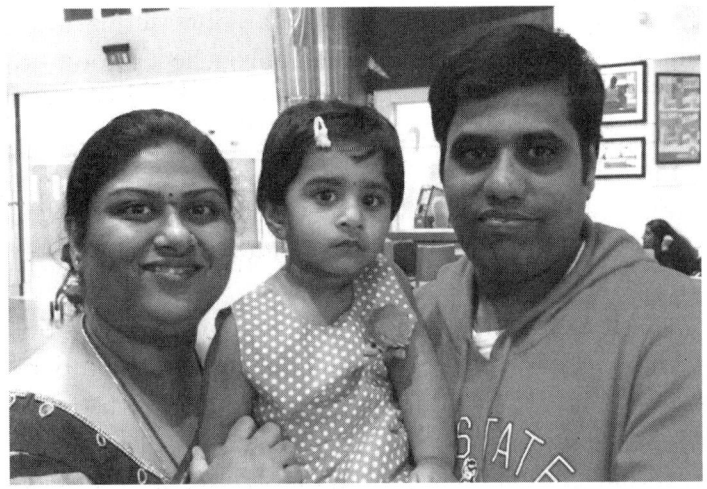

latest science, from psychology to biology, lay emphasis on learning even before being born. The nine-month period a baby spends in its mother's womb is not only for its physical and mental development but a lot of its learning takes place right there. This learning defines and shapes the baby for the rest of its life. Andal Madam has introduced us to the Talking to the baby in the womb concept when we were getting fertility treatment at her clinic. As soon as Sridevi became pregnant, we put this into practice. We spoke to the baby in the womb like we would speak to a friend. We talked to the baby about our dreams for her and about our daily routine. We read stories and sang songs to her in the womb.

Today we are seeing the benefit of the Talking to the baby in the womb technique. Unlike the other kids of her age, she likes sharing her toys. She is well behaved and a quick learner. Thanks to Andal Madam for her support and guidance throughout this amazing Talking to the baby in the womb journey.

Dr Andal has given a boon to all pregnant women in the form of the technique of Talking to the Baby in the Womb, I feel every pregnant mother and to-be mother must know this. As a person benefitted from this technique, to spread and share this to as many number of families as possible, its my privilege to lay strong foundation for a brave new world.

Doctor: It always gives me immense pleasure, to hear the journey of motherhood from the couple. I'm sure their stories will give happiness, hope, motivation and inspiration.

Dear Readers,

So far, I had been talking to you through Sahana. It was an enjoyable and enriching experience of sharing my journey of learning and evolving. Yes, from just an obstetrician conducting deliveries, I have grown into a catalyst of motivating mothers to offer a good child to the family and society through Talking to the Baby in the Womb technique. I deem it a great opportunity and blessing to closely observe the wonders of nature from conception to delivery, and not only a witness but also coordinate and play an active role in the miraculous event called birth. Though pregnancy is a natural process, it can at times be riddled with risk for the mother and the baby. Sometimes it is a cakewalk and sometimes there are moments of tightrope walking.

I feel blessed to learn the language of mind-body connection during pregnancy and delivery.

These events are controlled by hormones that depend on our emotional status. I started slowly understanding the meaning of the quote, 'the true medicine for disease is love.' Yes, I see lack of love in the form of anxiety and worry, causing miscarriages to hypertension during pregnancy, making advanced technology and ultra-modern treatment facilities fail in some cases. (Yes! Our medicines are not fear killers!) In some cases, along with medicine, the power of love in the form of reassurance from the family and doctor works wonders. To make the best use of technology and treatment, we need to practice reassurance and instil confidence and trust in expectant mothers. If taking treatment is like listening to a song, reassurance is like knowing the meaning of it, which makes the experience more effective. If eating food is treatment, the ambience and the hospitality are reassurance, making it a pleasant experience.

1) REGARDING DELIVERY:

We must know that though delivery is a natural process, sometimes a caesarean section becomes inevitable to safeguard the health of the mother and baby. We need to accept timely a caesarean section as a boon for the baby's well-being. If the baby's health is compromised, then even if it is normal delivery, it will not have served the purpose. Our primary goal is healthy and happy mother and baby, the mode of delivery is secondary. Nobody will remember or ask about the mode of delivery after a month, but optimal health of the baby and mother is necessary for personal and social reasons. We need to remember that delivery is a hormone-controlled event; if we give up goal-oriented anxiety, it can ensure smooth and easy normal delivery, provided other factors such as the baby's weight and position, heart-rate and well-being and maternal passage are normal. The role of an empathizing and reassuring birth companion can never be underestimated; he or she makes labour and delivery easy and bearable, sometimes even enjoyable and memorable. So, finally I ask the expecting mother and her family to be mentally and physically prepared for a normal delivery and wholeheartedly accept caesarean section if the situation warrants.

I have talked enough about the effect of 'Talking to the Baby in the Womb' on various aspects. Keep the goal of pregnancy as healthy and happy mother and baby. Let us remember to offer a memorable womb experience to the baby, which would no doubt lay the strong foundation for the rest of life. For that, we need to take a firm decision of not worrying about petty, short-term things and get sidetracked from having happy and quality time with the baby, making pregnancy and delivery healthy and treatment most effective.

2) SPREAD OF TALKING TO THE BABY IN THE WOMB

After reflecting on the impact of Talking to the Baby in the Womb on the child, I strongly feel that like-minded people must join hands to motivate the expectant mothers to produce a new generation of children with core values of great character, integrity, intelligence and success and prosperity with family bonding. We know the origin of Talking to the Baby in the Womb is in India with iconic figures of the Puranas, such as Prahalada and Abhimanyu. The recent past has shown us the line of continuity in Shivaji Maharaj and Swami Vivekananda of how their mothers' thoughts before and during pregnancy shaped their personality. We see this effect happen at a country level in Israel, where the people sow the seeds of intelligence during pregnancy. In our country, behaviour moulding was done during the freedom struggle, and great leaders were born in different parts of the country, such as Bhagat Singh, Lala Lajpat Rai, Mahatma Gandhi, Sardar Vallabhbhai Patel, V.O. Chidambaram, Veerapandiya Kattabomman and Subhash Chandra Bose. The absence of leaders of such calibre after Independence reflects the paradigm shift in the thinking pattern of society.

Present-day society gives importance to education, wealth and power. Mothers also dream of getting their children well educated and well settled. The result is increase in the literacy rate, trade and industrial development, and consequently improvement in the standard of living. Society, including expectant mothers, does not think of the other side of the coin, namely, moral values, character, personality and ethics, as an important part of success. So there is increase in selfishness causing unrest and violence in society. Our social life is glorious but personal life is miserable. The present scenario clearly shows that education gives only comfort and luxury and not happiness, security and peace. Why, in yesteryears, in spite of poverty and illiteracy, peace and security prevailed in society, and in the present day, on the other hand, unrest, violence and crime rates are increasing in spite of education, wealth and power. In the pursuit of power, we have marginalized the joint family system.

ROLE OF JOINT FAMILY SYSTEM

The joint family system had a tremendous impact on both the family and society and ensured their progress by passing on traditions, moral values and maintaining cultural integrity.

There was happiness in the family. There was peace in society.

FAMILY

It served as an effective emotional shock-absorber, giving a sense of security, emotional stability and happiness to every member of the family. Lack of strong interpersonal relationships has paved the way for increase of anxiety and depression.

SOCIETY

The continuation of the joint family system over centuries was the root cause for preservation of moral values and cultural practices. Those days, we used to love and respect people and follow ethics. Nowadays, we love material things and give less respect to people and ethics. The net result is the mushrooming of old-age homes, increase in the number of divorces and suicide rates. So the need of the hour is to modify the goal as success along with integrity and family bonding. Our missile man and spiritual scientist Abdul Kalam has the goal for us: 'Youth must be armed with technology and love for the nation. They must aim high.'

PAST:	Decrease in Literacy	→	Poverty
	Increase in MORALITY	→	Peace and security
	Increased family bonding	→	Happiness.
PRESENT:	Increased Literacy	→	Increased affluence, prosperity.
	Decreased moral values	→	Violence, insecure feeling.
	Decreased family bonding	→	Anxiety and depression.

SOLUTION

We cannot revive the joint family system, but we have to bring back the spirit of family bonding and ethics. We can form small family circles at the workplace, friends groups, living areas (apartments, colonies, etc.). As an extension of such programme, we can utilize the opportunity to mould the baby using the Talking to the Baby in the Womb technique during pregnancy.

Pregnancy has two dimensions: Physical, like the well-being of the mother and the baby, various tests, scans, medications taken during pregnancy for the well-being of the mother and the baby along with the delivery process. The other dimension is the personality, character of the child which is shaped by its mother's thoughts. Mothers are advised to read good books, listen to good soulful music, visualize the qualities of their ancestors or great personalities they admire, such as Vivekananda and Mother Teresa. Of late, more and more mothers are focusing on only the first dimension, that is physical well-being of the mother and child, and have totally forgotten the personality, character and traits the child should have, which are in her control in the nine months of pregnancy.

The awareness has to be created that every mother in her nine months of pregnancy or even before pregnancy can strongly influence the personality (quality) of the child by her thoughts irrespective of her educational standard (literate or illiterate), financial status(rich or poor), caste, colour, creed, religion or nationality.

I wish all the readers and their well-wishers a happy reading time along with health, happiness and abundance. I call upon people from all walks of life with a burning desire to motivate present and future mothers to dream of new-age children with success rooted in integrity and family bonding. Success gives happiness only when shared with others, and success based on integrity gives lasting happiness. Thus family bonding and integrity act as grease for the smooth functioning of the wheel of success. If this dream comes true, national and global peace and prosperity can be restored.

Jai Hind!

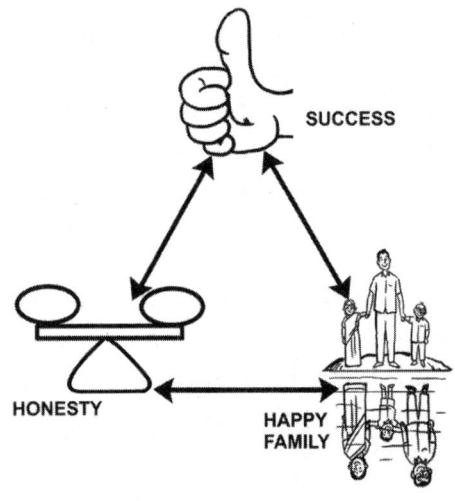